James Withey is the author of the bestselling books *How to Tell Depression to Piss Off: 40 Ways to Get Your Life Back*, *How to Tell Anxiety to Sod Off: 40 Ways to Get Your Life Back*, *How to Get to Grips with Grief: 40 Ways to Manage the Unmanageable* and *How to Smash Stress: 40 Ways to Get Your Life Back*, and is the co-editor of *The Recovery Letters: Addressed to People Experiencing Depression* and *What I Do to Get Through: How to Run, Swim, Cycle, Sew, or Sing Your Way Through Depression*.

He is the founder of The Recovery Letters project which publishes online letters from people recovering from depression. James trained as a person-centred counsellor and worked in addiction, homelessness and mental health services. He manages a range of mental health issues including depression, anxiety and PTSD. He lives in Hove in the UK, with his husband and emotionally damaged rescue cats. You can find him at www.jameswithey.com.

Also by James Withey

How to Tell Depression to Piss Off
How to Tell Anxiety to Sod Off
How to Get to Grips with Grief
How to Smash Stress

How to Sort
Your Self-Esteem:

40 Ways to Improve Your
Confidence and Self-Worth

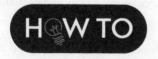

James Withey

ROBINSON

ROBINSON

First published in Great Britain in 2024 by Robinson

1 3 5 7 9 10 8 6 4 2

Copyright © James Withey, 2024
Illustrations by David Andrassy

The moral right of the author has been asserted.

Important Note
This book is not intended as a substitute for medical advice or treatment.
Any person with a condition requiring medical attention should consult a
qualified medical practitioner or suitable therapist.

A CIP catalogue record for this book is available from the British Library.

ISBN: 978-1-47214-911-4

Typeset in Sentinel by Initial Typesetting Services, Edinburgh
Printed and bound in Great Britain by Clays Ltd, Elcograf S.p.A.

Papers used by Robinson are from well-managed forests and other responsible sources.

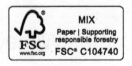

Robinson
An imprint of
Little, Brown Book Group
Carmelite House
50 Victoria Embankment
London EC4Y 0DZ

An Hachette UK Company
www.hachette.co.uk

www.littlebrown.co.uk

How To Books are published by Robinson, an imprint of
Little, Brown Book Group. We welcome proposals from
authors who have first-hand experience of their subjects.
Please set out the aims of your book, its target market
and its suggested contents in an email to
howto@littlebrown.co.uk.

To Michelle and Fi M

Contents

Introduction

Low self-esteem is a lying, thieving, hideous bully.

Everyone I know suffers from low self-esteem in some form. Well, to be fair, my cat thinks he's the bee's knees, so let's not count narcissistic felines, but everyone else. That's a lot of people not feeling good about themselves.

I don't remember a time when I didn't feel bad about myself. I always thought I wasn't clever enough, sporty enough, attractive enough, sophisticated enough or popular enough. I always thought that other people were better than me. I really didn't want to be me, I looked at others and wished I could be them. I spent years really hating myself and it caused so many problems along the way.

With low self-esteem we might experience depression, anxiety, loneliness or stress. It can cause problems in our romantic relationships, friendships, family and work life. We can develop unhealthy habits like drinking too much, eating disorders, smoking or other addictions.

We miss opportunities when we have low self-esteem;

1

we don't take chances, we shrink into ourselves because we don't think we have a place in the world. It can take everything from us.

It's a horrid, vicious cycle because when we tell ourselves continually we're worthless, we start to believe it even more. We become worthless because of what we are telling ourselves.

We have to break this spiral. We need to get this sorted because low self-esteem stops you from living fully; instead you are just existing. It's a waste of your life and, frankly, I've had enough and I hope you feel that you've had enough too. It's been running your life, but now is the time to take charge.

What we need is the tools to know how to raise our self-esteem to where it should be. We're going to change how you feel so that you live a wonderful, meaningful life knowing how bloody awesome you really are.

In this book we'll cover self-esteem and confidence. What's the difference, I hear you cry? Well, thank you very much for asking. Self-esteem is how we feel about ourselves looking inwards, i.e. our self-worth. Confidence is how we feel when we present ourselves to the world, i.e. what other people see. One impacts on the other, so the tips in this book work for both. It's a 'two for the price of one' kind of thingy – good, eh?

You can start anywhere in this book: you don't need to

go from page one. You can dip in and out, start at the back or the front if you want. I also give you permission to circle passages, highlight sentences that mean something to you. It's your book so use it how you need to. If I ever come to your house and check your bookshelves – which sounds a bit creepy to be fair – I want to see this book well-thumbed and written on. You can also write down things like 'My goodness, James is such a genius' and 'I really think James is a total guru and should be canonised as a saint.'

3

The book is short and has short chapters for a reason, not because I didn't have much to say, because I can talk about self-esteem and confidence for hours – you don't want to get me started in a pub with a gin and tonic, honestly. It's because when we feel bad about ourselves, our attention span is impacted, so a six-hundred-page book with charts, theories and tiny writing is going to feel massively intimidating. Also, I'll use some humour to make it easier to read. I mean, who wants to read a depressing six-hundred-page book, eh? Not me.

My advice is to read this book twice. I know, I know – but the thing is, on the second reading you will notice stuff that you didn't clock the first time around. And it's a small book, each tiny, weeny, itsy bity chapter will take a maximum of 3.597 minutes to read. Also, when people ask, 'Have you read this marvellous, multi-award-winning, internationally acclaimed book called *How to Sort Your*

Self-Esteem?' you can haughtily reply, 'Well, actually, I've read it twice.'

Also, like most things in life it takes a bit of work to sort our self-esteem, but please know that we can fix it because I've done it. You just need tips, techniques and insights that work for you and that's what the book will give you.

Improving your self-esteem is best done like pruning a tree. Do it regularly and it's much easier than getting a huge ladder and trying to lop the whole thing down when it's completely out of control. Once you've read a chapter, try and implement it, practise it and you'll start to see a change.

Not every chapter will speak to you and that's abso-lutely fine. There are forty to try, so if one doesn't work so well, try another. The different techniques also work at different times and for different things so experiment and see which ones help.

Shall we get started? If you're not sat with a hot drink – go and get one. Oh and grab one of those gooey pastry things you can buy in the posh patisserie. If you don't have a posh patisserie near you, I will personally give you the money to head to La Patisserie Cyril in Paris and buy some, it's all part of the service.

And finally, remember no matter what anyone else says, no matter what you're currently feeling about yourself, you *are* enough, you really, really are.

James

1. Joe says, 'make a list'

Here's a conversation with my friend Joe. We're having overpriced lattes at some achingly cool coffee shop, which we're clearly not cool enough to be in. The three baristas are about thirteen and called Magnolia, Waterfall and Pinecone. The cups are recycled organic baby food jars and I've cut the long conversation about how no one should pay the equivalent of three bags of gold for some caffeine, and no one is called Joe or James anymore.

> JOE: So, besides your hatred for baristas with nature-inspired first names, how are you?
>
> ME: Pretty much hating myself, loathing every single sinew, every character flaw, regretting every mistake I've ever made and realising I am utterly and completely worthless.
>
> JOE: Right, well excellent. So, I'm guessing changing your name to Moonflower isn't going to help?
>
> ME: Oh, shut up. Listen, how do you do it? You're

always Mr 'I love myself' without coming across like an arrogant banana.

JOE: Well, firstly, thanks so much for the compliment and secondly it takes some work.

ME: Why?

JOE: Because we're naturally programmed to be able to come up with a list of stuff that we hate about ourselves—

ME: —I'm a pushover. I don't set firm enough bound-aries. I'm too sensitive. I'm ugly. I make too many mistakes—

JOE: Okay, okay – enough, Moonflower. I think you've just proven my point. I was about to say, before you rudely interrupted, that we can easily come up with a list of things we hate about ourselves but not a list of things we like about ourselves.

ME: Ummm . . . okay – errr . . . well . . . I quite like my feet.

JOE: Your feet? Seriously? Do you? I mean they're a bit gnarly, wouldn't you say?

ME: Thanks. Now I have nothing.

JOE: My point is that unless we balance things out and really think about our good bits, we can be stuck in an endless cycle of hating ourselves and building a bigger and bigger list.

ME: And that lowers our self-esteem?

JOE: You catch on fast, Moonflower.

ME: So, what? I should make a list?

JOE: Yep, but best to do it with someone else if you can. You can do it by yourself too, it just takes a bit more time.

ME: Should I do it with you?

JOE: I think that's the direction this is going in, yes.

ME: Right, so . . .

JOE: You're still thinking about your feet, aren't you?

ME: I just think they're really pretty.

JOE: Okay, so apart from your obviously gorgeous tootsies, what else do you like about yourself?

ME: Ummm . . . I don't know. I don't like this game.

JOE: No one does, but that's why we need to do it because we spend all our lives criticising ourselves and not enough time giving major props to our good thangs.

ME: Sorry, did you just use the words 'props' and 'thangs'?

JOE: I did, one of the things I like about myself is my ability to play with modern vernacular. Stop distracting. Back to you, Moonflower.

ME: Fine, fine. I like that I have a sense of humour.

JOE: Right.

ME: I like that I care about others.

JOE: Does that mean you're going to pay for these stupidly expensive coffees?

ME: It does not. Err . . . I like how I fight for injustices. I like my passions, my interest in art, books and stuff.

JOE: 'Stuff'?

ME: I can't think of anything else.

JOE: Not a bad start, I guess. Now we write them down on a piece of paper.

ME: Can I do this on my phone as I don't have a spare eagle quill and parchment to hand?

JOE: You can. Now, what we do is build on that list, keep adding and keep looking at it, especially when you start thinking that you're a numbskull. It's a progressive aide-memoire.

ME: A whatty what what?

JOE: An active list, you ignoramus. It's not one of those that you do and just forget about, it's part of the building blocks to feeling better about yourself.

ME: Okay, I get it. Thank you.

JOE: You're welcome.

ME: You're going to keep calling me Moonflower forever, aren't you?

JOE: Yes, yes I am.

I realised that I'd spent all my life not thinking about the good parts of me. I minimised praise at work, 'Oh it was mostly an accident that I wrote that well received report.' I brushed off compliments from friends. 'Well, thank you for saying I'm a good listener but I'm really not.' I didn't absorb the positive feedback I got and never made an active list of the positive things about me.

My 'crap things about me' list was so much easier to write, and it still rumbles around in my head – we can't get rid of it altogether. But that's when I bring out the other list, Joe's list I call it, which is easier than saying 'progressive aide-memoire'.

I think you can guess I am going to ask you to do a list, because otherwise it will just be me doing it and that's like, completely unfair, but it's also a great step to sorting your self-esteem.

Now, it IS going to feel weird, I promise you that. It will feel like you're bragging and being an arrogant fool. You'll want to hide behind your hands with the sheer cringeworthy nature of this, BUT please, please, please, please continue.

I will show you my list again as it might make it easier to start afterwards. Also, don't worry if you only have a few items on your list – hey, getting one point on the list is a huge achievement when you have low self-esteem, or no self-esteem. It's all about building on that list, looking at that list and reminding yourself of it.

Joe's list

* I like my sense of humour
* I like that I care about others
* I like my hobbies and passions
* I like that I fight for injustice
* I like my feet

10   See that's not a bad start, eh? And then over time I have
built on it when I recognise things that I like about myself.

* I like that I've fought for my accomplishments
* I like my courage
* I like my tenacity
* I still like my feet

Right, now go write your Joe list and I mean actually go
and do it. Now. Don't just go and get the dinner ready –
your family or the dog or rabbit can wait, the rest of the
book can wait; this really can't. I'm sitting waiting for you
to do it. Don't disappoint me now . . .

Oh, and have a look at your own feet, they're really
delightful.

2. Try not to care quite as much (and wear some chain mail)

I get wounded easily and I'm not just talking about when my friend's dog attacks my arm because he's mistaken me for a squirrel, which he constantly does. When people say nasty things to me, directly or indirectly, I feel hurt.

Now some would call this being overly sensitive, as if that's a bad thing, or a snowflake, which are beautiful ethereal things, so I'm taking that as a compliment. The bottom line is, what others say can make us feel worse about ourselves and those of us with self-esteem issues tend to get wounded more easily.

When someone looks at me and goes, 'Oh gosh, James. Yes, you're looking so . . . *well*, aren't you?' I know they're saying I've put on weight and look worse than I did. When someone tells me 'You've always been quite chatty, haven't you?', it makes me wonder if I've spent my life gossiping.

And, of course, there are some incidents where people call me a 'pathetic pompous arse wipe', which, you know, doesn't need a lot of interpretation and is simply, completely untrue. So there.

It's not as easy as just going, 'Oh, nasty things don't hurt me anymore' and then getting on with making a decent fist at a sourdough starter, it just doesn't work like that. When someone shouts at us, a loved one is annoyed with us, it's hard just to go 'meh' and for it not to impact our self-esteem. Trust me, I've tried the 'meh' method and I'm here to tell you it doesn't make a bit of difference.

So, let's unpack why people say nasty stuff. Rarely do you find that someone, out of the blue, just as you're passing the bakers, comes up to you and tells you what a despicable person you are. Think about that for a bit. That never happens, does it? You see, there is *always* context to nasty comments, there are always reasons why people say this stuff.

Take the person telling me that I'm looking 'well', i.e. I've put on weight. Why are they saying this? It's unlikely to be a genuine concern for my health, otherwise they wouldn't phrase it like that. It's because *they're* worried about putting on weight themselves and having a dig at me is a way to try and make themselves feel better. Get me, amateur psychologist, eh? But it's totally true.

The person telling me I'm 'chatty' may think I talk too much but also no doubt thinks *they* gossip too much. And the person who shouted at me on my bike yesterday is probably pissed off because other cyclists have annoyed them in the past and if you're reading this, sir, I think you'll find I was riding perfectly safely – so there.

Hurtful comments are pretty much always about the person saying them and much less about you. Context, you see? There is always context. Bear that in mind when the hurtful stuff comes at you, because once we understand this it's then easier for our self-esteem not to be impacted.

13

Next, I'm going to get you to put on some chain mail. Bear with me, this will make sense, I promise. The thing about chain mail is it's great for not getting stabbed by a medieval broadsword but it's also great for knocking back potentially hurtful comments. Not literally of course, if you get called a 'deranged goblin' at a battle reenactment in Corroy-le-Château, Belgium, wearing your chain mail won't ping the words back. We're talking imaginary chain mail, which, you'll be pleased to know, is much easier to put on.

The thing about this imaginary chain mail is it repels all the bad stuff but lets you absorb all the good stuff. It protects your self-esteem and boosts it at the same time. Utterly marvellous. All we do is imagine we're wearing our repelling chain mail.

When someone shouts at me on the train for daring to want to sit where their precious bag is, I employ the chain mail and – *WHACK!* – it bounces off – hooray! When an acquaintance tells me my new shoes don't suit me at all, I employ the chain mail and – *POW!* – it bounces off – hurrah! When a colleague says they don't like my presentation which I've taken hours to prepare, I employ the chain mail and – *BOSH!* – it bounces off – whoopee! You hear the comments, but they're just comments that fly into the chain mail, they're no longer hurtful.

But when someone says they think you're a patient and kind person, it gets through the chain mail and makes you feel great about yourself.

The good stuff gets in, the bad stuff pings off.

Right, let's go to battle.

3. That feeling of meaning

Many moons ago, when I was a depressed teenager, I volunteered in a charity shop every Saturday for about four years.

Not the usual activity for an adolescent, I grant you. No long lie-ins for me, grumpily descending the stairs at twelve o'clock and spilling cereal all over the kitchen floor. No hanging around skate parks and drinking cheap cider on the beach – no wait, hang on, I may have done the latter. Anyway, my point is at eight o'clock every Saturday morning I was up and at 'em, walking into town to volunteer alongside a wonderful bunch of women, who were all at least sixty years older than me.

I wasn't allowed to be on the tills, you understand, that exclusive privilege was reserved for the truly experienced volunteers who knew about customer service and how to upsell a pair of faded corduroy hotpants. My skills were best served upstairs, sorting through the donations, checking for holes in pairs of knickers (yes, people used to donate old underwear), looking through books on how to flourish without a gall bladder, examining a porcelain figure of a frog dressed as Bo Peep. The work was always plentiful, bag after bag. As we sorted, we chatted, had cups of tea and put the world to rights.

After a while, I started to feel better about myself. I felt that I had some purpose and worth because, hopefully due to my volunteering, somewhere along the line, in a country that I'd only ever seen in my blue 1982 World School Atlas, someone was getting some food or tools or something to make their life easier. In a very small way, I'd helped with that.

When we do nice things for other people, we feel good about ourselves. When we do nice things for other people, we feel better. It makes us feel useful, worthy and valued. It feels like our lives have meaning and having meaning in our lives is absolutely crucial to our self-esteem. When there is no meaning in our lives, we feel bad about ourselves.

When I think back to my time working in the charity shop, it still makes me feel like a good person, plus I got a staff discount on a series of long duffel coats and a very interesting book about gall bladders, so there's that too.

You don't need to go and work in a charity shop, although I'm sure they'd be grateful for your help. We can do loads of other smaller stuff day to day. Pick up someone's wallet which has dropped in the street, smile at the tired shop assistant, email the nurses from your hospital appointment and tell them what a great job they did when your gall bladder was removed, bring some cat food into the animal shelter. Small acts of niceness work as well, but I'd really recommend doing something ongoing to make a bigger difference to your self-esteem.

Someone I know spends a lot of his free time knitting hats for premature babies in intensive care. He loves that he can contribute to keeping a baby alive, especially as he can't have children of his own. That act keeps him going in so many ways. He gets a thank you card from the hospital and has been down to visit the unit and see the babies wearing his hats. It's a beautiful thing and one of the ways he keeps his self-esteem raised.

Another friend volunteers on an allotment for people with additional needs. They plant seeds, weed, make compost, harvest the potatoes and pick flowers in the summer. She loves the mix of horticulture and help – combining her love of gardening and her passion for empowering others.

My cats were born in Romania. They were street kittens who were rescued and were brought over in a van with lots of other cats and dogs who needed homes. I look at them, destroying my sofa with their claws, waking us up at four o'clock in the morning, drooling over my laptop and think, well, I did a good thing there. They're not on the streets hunting for food anymore, they're being looked after and that brings meaning to my life and makes me feel better about myself.

We want to feel useful, we want to feel that our lives have a purpose. That feeling of meaning raises our self-esteem.

4. Affirmations – but not in a cheesy way

Please find a red velvet tasselled cushion, sit cross-legged in front of a mirror, smile broadly and repeat these words.

'I am gorgeous. I am beautiful. I am heaven sent from somewhere like heaven that is heavenly. I am radiant and talented and curious. I am intelligent; my cleverness shines through like a big bright shiny thingy. I am special, there is no one like me, I am me and there is no one akin to me, who is me. I rock. I give to others, I give to dogs and horses and tortoises and European water voles. I am a god of compassion. I am a role model to every living thing. I am a giver, a gifter, a people-enhancer. I have achieved amazing things, wondrous things, I have achieved even more than much more worthy and more beautiful people have achieved. I have created and smelt and embraced all the dazzlement that is my divine essence. Above all, I am unfailingly modest.'

Repeat this three times an hour each day whilst drinking a cup of you.

There's a lot of talk about affirmations these days. A LOT. I'm not going to suggest that you do anything similar to the above because this will induce permanent nausea and I wouldn't want that for you. We are going to do something like it, but I'm absolutely not calling it affirmations because if I did, I would have to run around my local park with my hands over my ears screaming, 'No, no, no!'

I was once at a team building day with work. Before I continue with this story, those three words, 'team building day', are enough to bring me out in hives and make me run for the hills. Anyway, I was sitting in a circle having just done an exercise where we had to knit our connections to each other using wool. As you can imagine, this exercise didn't go well because none of us could knit, so we spent the hour stabbing ourselves in the stomach with the needles and swearing under our breath.

In the next exercise we had to say nice things about each other. (I'm sure it was more complicated than that, but the trauma of the knitting has obliterated my memory.) Each person chose a colleague to say something nice to and, yes, if I really cast my mind back and squint with pain, there may have been a talking stick. When it came to my turn, I selected someone, said they were kind and thought the worst was over. Except I'd forgotten that someone had to say a nice thing about me in return. My co-worker looked at me and said:

'I'm really grateful to James. He's thoughtful, he always asks me how my day is going, and I've really appreciated that since my marriage broke up. He's been a real support above and beyond what you'd expect from a colleague. I'm proud to call him my friend.'

My heart seemed to falter. For all my blistering cynicism about this day I didn't expect there to be a moment that actually touched me, made me feel better and valued and worthy. I was embarrassed, obviously, because anything remotely complimentary always embarrasses me, but it also felt good. Really good.

I want you to think about a moment like that when someone has said something nice to you. It might be a small, off-the-cuff comment, it may have been more profound like my experience above. It's that warm, fuzzy, lovely feeling that I want you to concentrate on for a moment because we're going to try and get that feeling by saying to ourselves, 'I'm alright.'

'What?' I hear you cry. 'How in God's talking stick is that going to work, James?' Well, the thing is there's a process to go through. Importantly, note that I said *alright* – not 'I love myself', not 'I'm a magnificent human', just I'm alright. When working on self-esteem you can't just go from 'I hate myself' to 'I adore each fibre of my

21

body' in one simple step, despite what some wellness guru or influencer idiot tells you on social media.

So, we're going to start with 'I'm alright'. Simply that, nothing more, just 'I'm alright'. I want you to say it to yourself once a day for a month. Put a daily alert on your phone. Remember, nothing more nothing less, just say to yourself 'I'm alright'. You don't need to do it in front of a mirror or anything, there's no need for a velvet cushion – it will just take a second out of your day. Keep saying it even if you don't believe it. 'I'm alright.'

What might happen is that you'll get an intrusive thought going 'I'm not okay, I'm a piece of penguin poo.' That's okay, that's what's supposed to happen when you have low self-esteem. What I want you to do is, acknowledge that thought and say, 'Oh just sod off.' You can stick your tongue out if you want to and then just go back to saying, 'I'm alright.'

Then you build it up, but only do this *after* you've read this book. That's an order. So there. This is your chart for how you're going to progress in stages each month and what you're going to say.

Month one: I'm alright

Month two: I'm fine

Month three: I'm a good person

These statements to yourself don't disguise the fact that we're all flawed, we all make mistakes, sometimes we shout at the kids when they spill the milk, sometimes we wish ill on others because they've pushed in front of us in the supermarket. But if the statement went, 'I am flawed, I make mistakes, I shout at the kids, I wish ill on people in the supermarket, but I'm alright' then the focus is too much on the negative and not the positive and it's the positive that needs building. We're very accomplished at knowing our negative points so there's no need to focus on them.

If getting to 'I'm a good person' seems unattainable, that's completely fine. Just stick to 'I'm alright' for longer and when it feels right, move on to the next stage.

After a while, the fuzzy feeling of telling yourself that you're alright will increase. Keep noticing that fuzzy feeling. Keep saying the statements and, for goodness' sake, have an éclair as a reward.

Remember, your biggest achievement in life will be going from 'I hate myself' to thinking 'I'm alright.'

No exaggeration.

You can get your Harvard MBA or your first-class degree in Experimental Zoology from Cambridge and it will be nothing in comparison. I'm quite serious.

Finally, I'm here to tell you that I think I'm alright and I'm a good person.

23

5. Be okay with buggering things up

I once had to massage a six-foot seven Argentinian wizard.
When you woke up, you didn't think you'd be reading that
sentence today, now did you?

I really don't know how I get into these situations. I
was at a new agey men's wellness day in a local church
hall, which I thought would give me a chance to look at
some of my many, many, many issues (please email for a
sixty-four-page PDF copy of them should you wish to see
the entire list). But there was far too much drumming and
pretending to be a golden eagle for any useful work to be
done.

We were all in a circle and the person to my right was
massaging me – and doing a damn fine job actually – while
I was massaging a lovely man called Gordo on my left, who
told me he was a wizard from Cabo San Pablo in Tierra
del Fuego. Goodness knows what he was doing in my local
church hall. I suppose when you're a wizard you can travel

across hemispheres with a quick flick of your wand. He had a magnificent full-length beard and was wearing long purple wizard robes which, and I bet you didn't know this, are actually very difficult to massage through. At least that was my excuse because it became clear that I am not a good masseur.

Gordo tried unsuccessfully to disguise his wincing with a grimaced smile and looked back at me with encouragement, but it was clear he had never been in such pain in his entire life.

25

I had buggered it up. I was not going to become a professional masseur and set up my own flourishing shiatsu business, which was probably a good thing because until a few years ago I thought this was a type of Japanese dog.

You can go two ways when you bugger things up. You can go with stupid option one of beating yourself up every passing minute, telling yourself that you're a despicable person who is no good for anything and always gets things wrong. Or you can look at it a bit differently, so your self-esteem doesn't plummet even lower than the Pink See-Through Fantasia, which is a sea cucumber that lives way down in the depths of the ocean, and, for your delight, its anus and intestines are visible – so that's nice, eh? And there's another sentence you weren't expecting this morning.

I have a technique for this, it's secret option two: you don't beat yourself up. Radical, isn't it? I am a genius.

Okay, clearly it's not as easy as that, but, let me tell you, it's perfectly doable with practice. The trick is you have to catch yourself doing this really, really, really quickly, a sort of snatch and grab motion – like a wrestler.

I'll get something wrong at work, something that I'm used to doing all the time and the moment I realise I've got it wrong I'll start to go red, the embarrassment will take over and then the negative stuff will kick in. But before that happens, I jump in and go 'Noooooooooooo!' And then I'll remember that we all make frigging mistakes, every single one of us. This does not equate to us being a bad person. It just doesn't.

I failed my maths exams three times. Three times, people. I also failed my driving test three times. I seem to love failing at stuff in threes. My first driving test I didn't wait for a bus to pass and it got a tiny little bit near the car, the second test a huge lorry knocked a branch off a tree and it fell on the bonnet of my car – I was supposed to stop and assess damage or something – and the third time I forgot you had to stop at roundabouts. All very minor things, obviously.

I really, really wanted to pass my test the first time, I wanted it to be perfect. Those of us with low self-esteem are often massive perfectionists as well and I've learned that wanting everything to go perfectly is a sure-fire way of lowering our self-esteem.

Because . . . **you have to become okay with buggering things up.**

Learning how to bounce back and not beating ourselves up when things go wrong is crucial to how we feel about ourselves. Things *will* go wrong no matter how much you try, and accepting that is crucial.

Don't put failures and mistakes down to being a bad person. This just isn't true. It's simply a part of life.

It's what we do with the failure, in terms of our esteem, that counts. When you fail, fail well, someone once said – probably some Roman emperor – but my take on that is 'Fail, but don't then tell yourself you're an awful person for failing' which may not look as good on a t-shirt or tattooed up your arm in Arabic, but makes much more sense.

27

6. Stop comparing yourself to others

I'm on the bus to work. The train drivers are on strike, so I have to get up at three thirty in the morning, cycle a hundred miles to another town and get on a replacement service that only goes fifteen miles an hour and stops in every passing hamlet just to check if anyone wants to get on.

Okay, I have to get up half an hour early and cycle into town along the seafront for fifteen minutes to get a bus, BUT it feels like a huge inconvenience and I'm not in the best of moods.

I get on the bus ahead of everyone else, sit at the front and watch people getting on because I'm too grumpy to read my book. 'He's better looking than me,' I say to myself as a man gets on. 'She's got way more style than I have,' I think as a woman goes up the stairs with a superb hat and effortless sophistication. 'They don't have my problems,' I ponder as a group of friends take the back seats, laughing. On and on this goes until a small fluffy white dog gets on and I think, 'It's got way more hair than I have,' which isn't difficult to be fair.

None of this, not one iota, not one tiny speck on a tiny thing that you can only see in one of those special micro-scopes in a laboratory, makes me feel better. It makes me feel worse about myself. Every comparison lowers my self-esteem further and further. Comparison is the thief of joy, as the saying goes, but it's also a really, really quick way to lower your self-esteem.

You see, however much I want to be the 'good looking' guy, I can't morph into him. I am absolutely sure if I wear the woman's hat, I'll look like an exuberant eighteenth-century fop. At the time of writing, I don't have the ability to transfer my brain into other people's so that I no longer have any problems.

The bus sets off and, after ten minutes, I finally manage to connect my Bluetooth earphones to my phone after accidentally blasting out ABBA's 'Dancing Queen' three times to the lower deck. I start thinking about why com-parisons are so damaging to our self-esteem.

I reflect back to my teenage years when I compared myself to my siblings and cousins who all achieved more in their exams and went to better universities. The thing is I was measuring my self-worth by the narrow system of academia, not by anything else. I wasn't comparing how well we could all paint a picture or express our emotions

29

or understand poetry or build a sandcastle. Just exams, so of course I felt bad.

This applies to other comparisons as well. If we spend our lives going, 'I'm not as attractive as that supermodel,' then we will continue to feel crap about ourselves. If we think 'I can't jump as high as an Olympic champion,' then we will always feel like a failure. If we look at a multi-billionaire's motor collection and think 'I'll never be able to afford even one of his cars,' then you'll always feel less worthy. See what I mean?

Our self-worth should never, ever be dependent on anything superficial like a car or good looks. There are models with enormous self-esteem issues. There are high jumpers with self-esteem issues. There are multi-billionaires with self-esteem issues – they just drive nice cars and if any are reading this book and want to give me one, that's absolutely fine.

As the bus let people on and off, it finally turned into the main road and approached my stop. I knew that ruminating about being someone else had been a colossal waste of time. I am me and you are you and that's what we have to work with.

I realised we must base our self-worth on who we are – our integrity, our intentions, our compassion, our honesty, our self-awareness, our humility, our values – not by anything else that's unachievable or meaningless.

7. Don't avoid, don't procrastinate, do buy a croissant

31

I'm going for an interview for an adult education course. God, I hate interviews. To be fair, I'm guessing no one actually enjoys them. I doubt there's some random guy in Santiago de Compostela going, 'I'm sooooo excited. I have an interview tomorrow and then there are three further rounds to go if I get through this first one. I can't wait.' This would all be in Spanish, obviously.

I'm sat with my husband, grinding my teeth and not eating my dinner, and he's trying to persuade me to go.

> ME: I don't think I should go. I'll just be floundering around like one of those flat fish. What are they called again? The ones that flounder?
>
> HIM: Sole? Plaice? Turbot? Halibut?
>
> ME: Flounders.

HIM: For goodness' sake. Listen, you won't be, stop being ridiculous.

ME: All my nerves will come out when I speak, I'll sound like a fourteen-year-old boy whose voice is unsuccessfully breaking. I'm not going to go.

HIM: Okay, don't go.

ME: But do you think I should go?

HIM: Yes.

ME: But what if it's awful?

HIM: Then it's awful, but at least you went.

ME: They'll hate me, won't they?

HIM: They won't.

ME: I think I'll just stay under the duvet all day with a hot chocolate and cuddle the cats.

HIM: Okay.

ME: But do you think I should go?

HIM: Yes.

ME: Maybe I will go.

HIM: Great.

ME: Or maybe I'll stay at home.

HIM: Well, that's your choice but you might be missing out.

ME: Missing out on what?

HIM: Getting into the course.

ME: Oh yeah. Maybe I will go then.

HIM: Brilliant.

>   *[four hours later]*

ME: Do you think I should go?

HIM: YES! *[Husband self-combusts]*

33

When you have low self-esteem and low self-confidence, it's really common to avoid and procrastinate. We over-think. We doubt ourselves. We don't go to the Christmas party. We avoid the application form that could result in a promotion. We can't decide if we want to move house.

The problem is, because we don't like ourselves, we don't trust our decisions. When we make choices that turn out to be wrong, it gives us more evidence of us being terrible people.

We have to stop this train of thought. *Pronto. Rápidamente. Velocemente.*

We stop this train of thought by reminding ourselves of the four statements that fairies have etched in tiny, tiny, tiny writing on each and every four leaf clover found at the end of a double rainbow.*

---

* This may not actually be true.

* I will try things, if it doesn't work out then at least I have tried
* I won't let fear stop me from doing things
* I will take safe risks on things that might give me a reward
* Nothing will go perfectly, that's not due to me being a bad person

34 When we take risks and make decisions, we need to congratulate ourselves, whether it works out or not. The famous quote goes 'A life lived in fear is a life half-lived', but actually a life lived in fear is a life *barely* lived.

I went to the interview and was given a place: all cause for celebration. But the big celebration had to be that I didn't let fear and my low self-esteem stop me from doing it. That's the big reward. So, I bought a croissant. And now every time I make a decision and take a risk, I buy a celebratory croissant. Please do the same.

8. Who said you were a bad person?

I'm thirteen and I'm in France for the first time on a school trip. I've eaten a particularly delicious tarte tatin, tried some meat that everyone says was horse, been amazed that the basic greetings I've learned in class actually work – this stunned me the most for some reason – and I've also had some really funky chewing gum.

Now we are all on a coach to some rural wastewater filtration facility. Why anyone thinks a group of teenagers would want to see this in the UK is beyond me, but to suggest it as an activity when we're in France is bizarre in the extreme. Is French sewage intrinsically more interesting than British sewage I wonder as we travel along. We'd all much rather wander aimlessly through a non descript town and buy chewing gum.

We stop for a toilet break at somewhere called Dull. As I get off, the ferocious Liverpudlian teacher asks me how I'd pronounce the name of the town, obviously trying to trip me up so she can laugh at my expense. I don't know what to say because I'm not sure how to say the word in French. I mean is it 'Doul' or 'Deull' or 'Deill' even? And now other children are behind me waiting to get off, so I just panic and say 'dull'. She looks at me, smiles that she's caught me in her trap and says, 'The thing about you, James, is that *you're* dull. Now get off the bus.'

This has always stayed with me. Ever since I've wondered if I *was* dull. Was I just a boring and insipid person? Maybe people were so bored of me they had to buy strange-flavoured chewing gum to relieve the sheer ennui of my stale presence?

Logically, in my adult head, I know that she was just provoking me. Using her power as a teacher to bully any child she chose for her own titillation, and it could just as easily have been the next person in the queue to get off the bus. But as a child this stuff is harder to process, **because you're a child.**

It's much, much harder when someone we love, value and care for tells us we're unworthy. Maybe your mother told you were bad and it really stung. We might have been told every day that we were unlovable by a grandparent. Maybe a brother always took the time to say how stupid we were. Maybe we were constantly abused by an uncle. It's hard to shake off those memories and the impact they have on us.

You see, we're all impacted by our childhood, it's impossible not to be. Now, I can hear a bunch of retired colonels from High Wycombe going, 'Just pull yourself together man and have a bit of backbone.' Well, screw you, sir, because the worst thing you can do for your self-esteem is to bottle everything up and not acknowledge the repercussions childhood has on you. But if you're reading this and you *are* a retired colonel from High Wycombe, I'm sure you're lovely really.

You see, we need certain conditions as a child – love, security and to feel that we are valued and significant. If any one of those isn't in place, then our self-esteem lowers and this can have profound consequences. As children, when we're hurt, we think it's our fault. We blame ourselves because we don't understand the wider context or a world beyond our own. This leads to shame and hate, it can be deep set and very damaging.

We need to sort through these messages so we can see the comments for what they are and stop them affecting us so much. It's like a big bowl of self-esteem wool we have to untangle.

Let's be very clear. Those messages we were told as kids come from people who didn't know any better. They said stuff in the heat of the moment without thinking. They said stuff because they didn't know how to care for children. They said stuff because they couldn't manage others' behaviour. They said stuff because they wanted to feel powerful. They said stuff because they were stressed. They said stuff without realising the long-term impact it was going to have. They said stuff because they were called the same when they were kids – because they too were hurt when they were young.

None of these are excuses. Absolutely not. It's just that having an explanation takes the truth and power out of what they said to us.

As a child I was repeatedly told that being gay was wrong. That gay people are abnormal, that gay people are inferior, that they're a genetic mutation that needs to be corrected. It profoundly affected my self-esteem. I grew up hating myself for being attracted to men. There was no one on television that was gay, no famous people came out, no one at school admitted they were gay. No one said it was okay. No one validated my feelings of being attracted to men.

When you keep hearing the same message over and over again, it's hard not to believe it. Now I understand that the people who were saying this to me lacked knowledge, were scared, were saying what their religion told them to or, you know, were just assholes.

Messages from wider society impact us and they can come from fellow children as well as adults. We might be told being disabled makes you less valid or being black or being trans is less worthy. If we get these messages, the impact is profound.

Applying logic really helps here. How can you call a child stupid when they're just a child? How can you say people are unlovable when they've barely started their life? It just doesn't make sense. We have to take the power out of those statements, because they're nonsense, and we're going to do that by summoning Mr Spock from *Star Trek*.

I don't know a lot about the TV programme except my husband is a fan of the one with Jean-Luc Picard, but I do know that Spock says 'illogical' a lot in the 1960s series, which is all you need to know really. You can search on the internet to see what he looks like as it's good to get a mental image.

When a negative childhood message pops into my head, Spock immediately teleports and says, 'Illogical, James, no child is unworthy.' Or 'James, that is illogical, because no child can be said to be useless.'

The Spock Method works, it just does. Spock says things like:

'No one is less valid because of their mental illness, that's illogical.'

'Because someone is different from the norm, it's illogical to say that they are less worthy.'

See how it works? When you talk to Spock, so many

things we were told when we were growing up don't make sense. You might have guessed already that I'm quite an emotional person, my thoughts and feelings go up and down, which impacts my self-esteem. Having Spock challenge my thoughts is so useful because he brings everything back to logic, which I often struggle with.

Spock also wants to remind you that you are an adult now, not a child. These messages that hurt you as a child can no longer damage you as an adult when we see them for what they are. The greatest response to those that have hurt us, is loving ourselves and living our lives.

Now, live long and prosper. (I'm doing that Vulcan hand gesture thingy.)

9. Give Buster some love

I'm in a counselling session, where, to be honest, I spend
quite a lot of my spare time. If I got reward points for
therapy, I would have enough to pay for my own solid gold
mindfulness meditation and relaxation spa resort in
Bora Bora.

Here's how the conversation went with my therapist
that day.

> THERAPIST: How much compassion do you have for
> yourself, James?
>
> ME: How much of the – what, sorry?
>
> THERAPIST: Compassion.
>
> ME: Oh, well, I have a monthly direct debit to a donkey
> sanctuary and I also give to—
>
> THERAPIST: No, no, self-compassion. Compassion for
> you, James.
>
> ME: Well, I enjoy a nice yoghurt every now and then.
> I don't know if you're familiar with a medium protein

mix of peach, papaya and guava, but, boy, does it hit the spot. And then, of course, there's the high-octane combo of Greek yoghurt infused with wild berries. If you add a warm spoon of twenty-year-old brandy, it is, in my opinion, better than any cold remedy there is on the market.

THERAPIST: Right. Fascinating. I'm just wondering, besides yoghurt, are there other ways you show yourself compassion?

ME: Besides yoghurt?

THERAPIST: Yes. If we take yoghurt completely out of the equation.

ME: Gosh.

THERAPIST: How do you forgive yourself? How do you unburden yourself? How do you show yourself kindness? Any ideas?

ME: *[I sit in silence for the next thirty minutes]* I can't think of anything, no.

Self-compassion is not the same as self-care, although it sounds similar. Self-compassion is being as nice to yourself as you are to other people. Unless you're horrible to other people, in which case this isn't going to work. It's about realising your worth and treating yourself with respect. It's about comforting yourself when things go wrong.

I want you to imagine a dog. His name is Buster, he's three years old and lives on the streets in Hungary. He has to find scraps in bins, sleep on the streets and constantly keep an eye out for other dogs who pinch his food. Sometimes people beat him for the hell of it, but occasionally people feed him sausages or pieces of meat from their sandwiches. Mostly he's starving.

I don't know about you, but I'm starting to cry a bit and it's not even a real dog. Anyway, you see a picture of Buster and decide to adopt him. When he arrives at your home, he needs a lot of love and patience. You have to look after him very carefully, give him love, tenderness and affection, understanding that he's been hurt in the past, knowing that he carries trauma with him and doesn't like himself.

And, yes, you may have guessed it by now, how you treat lovely Buster the dog is how I want you to treat yourself. How you talk to Buster is how I want you to talk to yourself. How you love Buster is how I want you to love yourself. How you forgive Buster for the occasional accidents on the sofa is how I want you to forgive yourself because self-compassion is the antidote to any shame we might be feeling.

It's all about correcting the harsh things we're saying and introducing kinder words, more understanding and much more love. It's about clocking when we're being hard on ourselves and thinking, 'Would I treat Buster this way?'

If the answer is no, then change your tone, change your words and change your attitude towards yourself to make it much more compassionate.

Self-compassion is about allowing yourself to live a full life.

Self-compassion is when you're not hating yourself.

Self-compassion is when you forgive yourself.

So, please, be gentle with yourself.

10. Rely on you

There is a very ancient saying from the north-east of
Svalbard which says, 'You are but a lowly albatross and
you must fly alone to become the truest bird of which you
seek.' Profound, eh?

Okay, I totally made that up, but some of it is true. If
we continually rely on reassurance and help from other
people, the message is that we can't be trusted to rely on
what *we* think of ourselves. Basically, we need to put the
brakes on getting validation from others and get better at
validating ourselves.

Fine, in theory, I hear you say, but how do we do that?
Well, let me tell you a tale. This one is not as old as time,
nor is it made up, you'll be glad to know.

A few years ago, I spent quite a lot of time clubbing,
hoping that I would find a nice boyfriend who I could settle
down with and combine book collections into a fully
fledged library. The trouble was, one of my friends who I
often went out with was a traditionally handsome young

buck about town and he got all the men I admired. Damn and blast his eyes!

I would spot a nice-looking chap and think, 'Oh, what a fine gentleman. He looks of good health and breeding. He could be husband material.' In my head I'm already planning a nice summer wedding with jaunty bunting, cascading peonies draping across white-lined trestle tables full of matching vintage crockery when – BOOM! – my friend would snatch him from under my nose. The rakish brute! If I could have challenged him to a duel at dawn with a cursory drop of my gold embroidered gauntlet, then I would have done so, but there's some sort of silly law against fighting to the death or something.

As you can imagine, this didn't do much for my self-esteem. With every man he snagged into his bed chamber, I grew to hate myself more and more. This was clearly a problem because my self-worth was being based on whether other people were attracted to me or him. If they liked my friend more, that meant I was unworthy. When you read it, it sounds ludicrous, doesn't it? But I suspect you have been in similar situations in your life when you let others dictate your self-worth.

Drumroll please . . . it's now time for a children's playground seesaw metaphor, I know you've been *dying* for one of those. On one side you've got people saying lovely things about you, on the other side we've got people saying negative things and you're in the middle. The trick is to try and limit the amount of seesawing (is that a word?) from side to side because this rocks your self-esteem too much.

Our plan is to try and keep your self-esteem steady and healthy and in the middle of the seesaw, by what YOU do, what YOU say to yourself, how YOU feel about yourself – not impacted by others too much. Does that make sense?

If people call you an atrociously arrogant pig's bladder, then you will move over to one side and if someone tells you that you have the good looks and glamorous demeanour of ancient Byzantium royalty you will go over to the other side.

We might think that nice compliments that make us feel like a hot, sexy potato are great for our self-esteem, but they will only take us so far; it's like the fast food, nice at the time but you can't live on it.

For more nutritious, long-lasting self-esteem, we have to get to know ourselves and rely on ourselves to boost our self-worth.

When we start to shift our focus away from other people's validation or invalidation of us and understand that we are inherently worthy no matter what people say, our self-esteem stabilises.

When we feel we need to seek reassurance from others to feel valued, I want you to say this mantra:

47

'I am worthy no matter what people think of me or say of me.'

Repeat this when you feel tipped from one side or the other on the seesaw and it will bring you back to the centre, knowing your intrinsic worth. Or in other words, it will restore your fabulousness.

11. Is that actually true?

You're in court, I'm afraid. Sorry about that. But fear not, 49
you've not been arrested for smuggling three thousand
kilos of popping candy across the Mexican border, you're
actually here because the judge is going to preside over
your self-esteem beliefs. That's a relief, isn't it?

You see, with low self-esteem, we often have beliefs
about ourselves that are nonsense and would never hold
up in court, including:

* I'm ugly
* I'm a bad person
* I'm lazy
* I'm a useless parent
* I'm a terrible friend
* I'm a useless cake baker

The last one is more about me admittedly, you don't want
to try my apple upside-down cake.

We have to challenge these beliefs to be able to sort our self-esteem. The judge is going to want clear, substantiated evidence and, honestly, we very rarely have that.

Let's see how some of my non-apple-upside-down-cake-related beliefs hold up and then you can have a go yourself. The judge, Dame Sabrina Esteem MBE, is presiding and she's going to use the phrase 'Is that actually true?' to test our beliefs. I want you to remember this phrase because you're going to use it in daily life when these beliefs crop up in your head.

'The next case, your honour, is James Withey, who believes he is a bad person.'

'Right, Mr Withey, you need to demonstrate beyond reasonable doubt that you are a bad person. I believe you are representing yourself, so you may proceed.'

'So, I just kinda *feel* like I'm a terrible person.'

Long silence.

'Is that it, Mr Withey?'

'Well, yes, okay. Wait, I know. I once had terrible thoughts about a colleague and wanted him to fall over – not to badly hurt himself, you understand, just so that he maybe grazed his knee because he was bullying other people and making them cry.'

'Those thoughts happen to most of us, Mr Withey. Anything else?'

'Errr . . . I'm not as kind as I should be.'

'And that makes you bad?'

'Umm . . . Oh, I know! I tend to forget people's birthdays, I don't mean to and it's not about not loving them, I just forget. And I once broke up with someone over the phone.'

'Mr Withey, you are in danger of wasting court time if you don't come up with clear evidence that you are a bad person.'

'No, hang on! I've got it, I've got it. As a child I accidentally dropped a puppy and it hurt its leg.'

'Mr Withey, are you responsible for the slaughter of millions of people?'

'I don't think so, no.'

'Has any divine being descended from the heavenly skies and presided on your inherent evil?'

'Not that I'm aware of, no. But, you know, I'm out at work a lot so they may have missed me and there was that time when I was having cheese on toast and felt a bit funny, so it could have been then.'

'Mr Withey, is it actually true that you're a bad person? Because you can't produce a single piece of evidence.'

'It may not be true, I guess. Sorry, your royal judge-ness, your honour, thank you so much.'

It's hard living in our own heads, isn't it? We get into muddles. We convince ourselves of things that aren't true. Using this method makes you look clearly at how you see yourself and makes you challenge whether it's true or not. If it's not true, then we need to ignore that thought.

We can use it for deep set beliefs, like being a bad person, or bad parent, but also for day-to-day thoughts, such as 'I delivered the presentation badly'. It challenges our automatic assumptions.

Unless we confront these thoughts, we end up believing what we're telling ourselves and if you continue to do that, I am going to have to send Dame Sabrina Esteem round your house to look down at you from her half-rimmed glasses – a truly terrifying thought.

So keep asking yourself, 'Is that actually true?'

12. Do uncomfortable stuff

I'm in a cave.

I really, really, really hate caves. Once I was on a school trip and the light on my helmet got stuck while I was trying to get through a gap in a cavern called The Letterbox and a teacher had to push me through. Since then, I have, understandably, been a bit averse to them.

But now, here I am walking through the floodlit passageways and loathing every second. At points you have to crouch down to get through, which makes me start to sweat. I ask the tour guide how long until the end. 'About half an hour' she says, at which point I ask if there is an escape hatch, but she doesn't know what I mean and so the only option is to keep going.

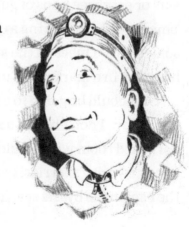

Everyone else is loving it. Taking photos, doing selfies

next to the stalactites or stalagmites – I don't know which they are and I really, really don't care. (Please don't email me to tell me what the difference is. One goes up, one goes down, blah, blah, blah.)

Why, you may ask, entirely reasonably, am I doing a long walk in some caves when I can't stand them? Well, because sometimes I like to get uncomfortable. It really helps my self-esteem. I suspect your brow is now furrowed and you're thinking, 'This man is a lunatic, why am I reading his book?' Another fair question.

You see, getting out of our comfort zone is incredibly helpful. When we do something that's out of our normal range of experiences, it gives us evidence of our worth. It tells us we are capable of exceeding the limits we place on ourselves. I kept telling myself I could never go in a cave again, but I did – I hated it, but I bloody well did it.

You don't need to trek through the Gobi Desert on skis or eat three kilos of guava in four minutes. It can be 'small' stuff, like asking a question at a conference, telling someone you meet on the street that you like their scarf, haggling in a market in Turkey.

Or it could be going to a silent disco. Which is what I did next. Now, I don't like to dance in front of anyone, even in a darkened room with music blaring and having consumed one or two dry sherries. I certainly don't like to dance on the esplanade by the sea, in sparkly flashing headphones, in front of the whole city, wearing my duffel coat. Yet, here I am, shuffling around like a dazed octopus to a selection of Elvis, Madonna and the Backstreet Boys.

Initially, I clock every passer-by and think, 'God, they're judging me, looking at my pathetic Elvis impersonation and seeing my feet flailing about like a drunk goose.' However, overall, I'm just grateful that I haven't fallen over yet.

Other people join the group and immediately start flailing their arms and legs around. They seem to have no inhibitions at all. After a while, I start to get a bit more confident. As songs that I love come on, I move a bit more and, to be honest, it also helps that it's getting dark. I was doing it – actually doing it. I hadn't gone and sulked by the bins, I hadn't given up and gone home, I was still dancing and one might almost say I was bustin' my best moves and, darn it, I was proud of myself.

You see, doing uncomfortable stuff makes you see you CAN achieve.

When we do this, it boosts us, it helps us to see we are more than our fears. We are *so* much more than who we think we are.

13. Forgive yourself for past mistakes and don't steal stationery

Sometimes we can feel haunted. Not by the ghost who roams the local churchyard ringing a hand bell every Michaelmas shouting, 'Be gone, ye stranger, there is only evil hither,' but by the things we did in the past that make us feel ashamed.

The thing about shame is that it really drags our self-esteem down, so we need to get a handle on it and start forgiving ourselves.

We all have things we're not proud of, times in the past that make us think, 'I can't believe I did that.' Maybe we broke up with someone in a less than perfect way. Maybe we regret not going to see that relative before they died. Maybe we didn't see enough of our children when they were growing up.

We can spend way too much time thinking about what we *should* have done and what we *didn't* do. This damages our self-esteem because the message to ourselves is 'I did something shameful therefore I'm a terrible person'.

I truly believe most of us aren't horrible people – apart from the people who invented squeezy Marmite, because you shouldn't mess with the sacred glass container – but I feel this may be just my issue. Oh, also, whoever decided to discontinue the Wispa chocolate bar, but, again, it's probably just me that needs to deal with this. And yes, I know they were reintroduced, but it still really hurts.

When I was younger, I had a job as a carer for a man who had physical disabilities and brain damage from a road traffic accident. I would go round each day, we would chat, usually do some quizzes or listen to music, and then I would help him get into bed. It was a great job, we got on well, but it was only for a few hours a day and after a while I had to get something different as I needed more money to pay the rent. I explained this to him, and he was sad I was leaving, but I promised that I would come back and visit him. And, yes, you've guessed it, I didn't go back. I know. I know.

Thinking about this makes me feel truly terrible. It makes me blush and mutter with shame. It makes me want to turn back time and make it right.

Would I do the same thing now? I really, really hope not, but just because I'm older doesn't mean I won't make mistakes. Hell, I make them all the frigging time, BUT this doesn't mean I'm a bad person; it just means I made a mistake.

When I look back at this I automatically think, 'What a selfish person you are. What an irresponsible person you are. What a cruel person you are.' But just read those comments back. I'm saying to myself 'I am a selfish, irresponsible and cruel person' and the thing is, and I don't want to boast here, but I just don't think that's true.

That's the crucial bit, folks. I made a mistake but I'm not inherently bad. See the difference? Our actions may have been misguided or selfish but that doesn't mean we are. You have to challenge these thoughts and you also need to forgive yourself.

Whilst we're confessing, I need to tell you that I once stole a pencil sharpener from my classroom when I was six. I'd like to apologise to Miss Plowman, who trusted me not to pinch stationery, and to my fellow pupils, who didn't realise they were at school with a master criminal. And, yes, I still feel bad about this.

This is going to be uncomfortable, but I want you to think about the times in your past when you did something you regretted, which still impacts on your self-esteem. Perhaps you passed on a secret after being told not to. Did you neglect a friendship that never recovered? We're not doing this to make you relive the guilt; it's about acknowledging the mistakes, but not taking it to the next level where it continues to impact you.

So, how do we forgive ourselves? Well, first by seeing that we're human and there's not a person on earth who's not made a mistake. Not Mother Teresa, not Florence Nightingale. Even Jesus shouldn't have overturned those tables in that market. Very unfair on the stallholders if you ask me.

When you see mistakes as part of being human and realise that it's impossible not to make them, then we can see our errors for what they are: regrettable, yes, but also inevitable as we all try and get through this strange thing called life.

Secondly, what's the purpose of holding on? If we've learned from them, seen that they were misjudgements, then letting them continue to impact on our self-worth is serving no purpose at all. It's time to let go. Say it again.

It's time to let go.

It's time to let go.

IT'S TIME TO LET GO.

I forgive my younger self, I really do. I obviously haven't turned into archangel Gabriel. Or the Prophet Muhammad. The last time I checked I'm not the reincarnation of Buddha, but I know that these events don't define me, can't define me, because if they do, I will continue on the path of self-destruction, hating myself more and more.

Now, I just have one small question to ask you. You can say no, of course, but can I borrow your pencil sharpener?

14. Core blimey beliefs

We all have a list of things that we believe about ourselves – values and behaviour that we need to uphold to feel good about who we are. The fancy schmanzy psychology name for them is core beliefs. I like to take a Mary Poppins point of view (well, more Bert the chimney sweep) and call them 'core blimey beliefs' (you have to do the bad cockney accent too), because it can surprise you when you take a closer look at what they are.

These beliefs develop from our experiences, our upbringing, our childhood; what our parents taught us or demonstrated to us, but also our opinions and views as we grow up and make sense of the world.

For your delectation, I present my list of core beliefs. If you have a spare bugle with you, please sound a fanfare now.

* I must work as hard as possible
* I must always think of others before myself
* I must always look youthful
* I must be on time

* I must always be polite
* I mustn't get angry
* I must be thin to feel attractive
* I must always be kind
* I must never be off sick from my job

When these core beliefs are compromised, you start to feel rubbish about yourself and your self-esteem plummets.

The trouble is, keeping up with these beliefs is basically impossible. Now, clearly, obviously, I'm a completely perfect human being and never diverge from this list, but my understanding is that you aren't? Is that right? I thought so.

In order to keep our self-esteem on an even keel, we have to change some of these core beliefs to something more realistic. More of that in a second. Firstly, I want you to write your list of core beliefs. Think about the message you received growing up and what standards you have about yourself and how you look and behave. Take a bit of time on this, I'll be here when you get back.

Done that? Yes? Excellent.

What we're going to work towards is an acceptance of imperfection. We're not going to beat ourselves up when we don't stick to our core beliefs, because and let's say it again for those at the back, nobody is perfect.

We're going to start with my list so you can see how it's done and then you can have a go with yours.

'I must work as hard as possible' changes to *I like to work as hard as possible, but it's not the end of the world if I don't.*

'I must always think of others before myself' changes to *I can think of others and myself, it's not one or the other.*

'I must always look youthful' changes to *Everyone ages, everything changes, we all get older, it's better to embrace this rather than chase youth which is fleeting. I'm okay the age I am now.*

63

'I must be on time' changes to *I prefer to be on time but there will be some times when I'm not and that's okay.*

'I must always be polite' changes to *It's important to me to respect others, but there will be times when I'm being disrespected or feel under threat, that I won't manage this.*

'I mustn't get angry' changes to *Everyone gets angry, it's a universal emotion and it's OK if I feel cross.*

'I must be thin to feel attractive' changes to *My self-worth is not dependent on how much I weigh or how I look.*

'I must always be kind' changes to *I like to be kind to others but there will be times when I'm not and I'm not a bad person if this happens.*

'I must never be off sick from my job' changes to *We all get ill and there will be times when I'm not well enough to go into work. That doesn't mean I'm going to lose my job or that I'm bad at my job.*

Do you see how we do it? Have a look at your list and see how you can change your core beliefs to something more realistic. Accept that you're not perfect.

Remember, when these core beliefs are compromised our self-esteem goes down. When we change them to something more realistic, our self-esteem stays on an even course.

15. Catch your catastrophising

Two days ago, I sent a message to my friend. I asked if they wanted to go and see a play in town in a few weeks' time. They haven't got back to me yet. Here I present what my low self-esteem brain has been saying:

Clearly, they hate me. They've decided that they no longer want to be my friend. Which is completely understandable, I mean who would want to be my mate? I wouldn't want to. It's probably because I was a day late saying happy birthday to them fifteen years ago and they have been secretly hating me ever since and just pretending to want to spend time with me. They're probably off with their other friends who they love more, who say happy birthday on time. You can't blame them for that. Should I send them another message? But then I will look really needy and that will be another reason not to be friends with me. Not that they need another reason, of course. I could send them another message saying that I fully understand they no longer want to be friends and wish them all the best with their other better friendships in the future. But then, if, by a very slim chance, there's a reason they've not got in touch, I will sound like a deranged hippo and then that *will* be a reason not to be friends with me.

When I'm out for lunch and someone says they have to leave early, I assume that they've had enough of my company. When someone says they're busy and can't meet up, I think they don't want to spend time with me. When someone ends a phone call early, I assume they have better things to do than to talk to me. We low self-esteemers *love* catastrophising.

It's exhausting, eh? We rush to think the worst about people and situations. Low self-esteem feeds catastrophic thoughts and paranoia.

When we think we're not good enough we assume that everyone also thinks we're not good enough. Because we hate ourselves, we just assume people hate us as much we do and that's rubbish.

The thing is, folks, it's not always about us. Here's the message I got back from my friend.

Hi James. Sorry not to have got back to you earlier. I had to take Ruby to the doctor as she scraped her knee in the park and it looked a bit weird. Then the dog decided to eat my slippers while I was wearing them, but yes, I'd love to go to the theatre! Andy has agreed to babysit, let's have some Thai food beforehand and catch up. Can't wait. xxx

I suddenly saw how ridiculous our self-esteem brains can be, thinking the worst, making suppositions, making assumptions.

If we let our self-esteem brain take control of our thinking, not only is it an emotional rollercoaster, it's also doing us a massive disservice. We have to think more logically and less emotionally when we start to catastrophise.

I do this by draining my self-esteem thoughts. I pour the thoughts into a sieve and what happens is the logic and reason get through, but it blocks the misguided emotions and I discard them. I then change my train of thought to something with more reason.

This is what my brain says to me when I catch and sieve my catastrophising:

I'm sure she's busy and will get back to me soon. If I don't hear from her in a few days, I'll message again to make sure she's okay. It's probably not because she doesn't like me because we often go to the theatre and she's happy to come.

What a difference. Night and day. One where emotion takes over and one where reason takes over.

Catch it, sieve it, sort it out.

67

16. Celebrate big styley

I'm waiting for my degree results.

The last four years have been a massive slog. In my first year, my mental health was horrendous. I felt suicidal a lot of the time, but this was circa 1823 so there was no support available, and the internet was just a distant idea in Tim Berners-Lee's brain.

I was adjusting to coming out as gay, with all the complications that involves. My first time in a gay club. Telling friends and family who I was. Then in my final year a close friend died suddenly of meningitis, which is what my dad died of. That's quite a list of crap stuff.

That's not the whole picture, of course. There have also been nights of dancing into the early morning; laughing until my lungs hurt; fabulous, boozy nights in cheap Italian restaurants; and sunny days lazing in parks reading books and having picnics.

Now, I'm about to walk into the room and find the piece of paper that will tell me whether I've passed my degree and, if so, what grade I've got. All the good bits and the bad bits of the last few years are rushing through my head, and I start to feel dizzy.

What if I've failed? What do I do then? All the studying, all the reading, (all the drinking), all the essay writing will have been for nothing. My friend asks me if I'm feeling okay. I tell him I need a chair. He gets one and I put my head between my legs – I don't know what this will achieve, but I've seen it in films so it must be the right thing to do.

One of the lecturers opens the door and lets us in. There's a mad rush with people eager to get to the front. I hear people scream with delight when they see how well they've done. Others slowly withdraw from the room with a rueful grin, hiding their disappointment.

The list is divided into grades so I start at the bottom with the passes – no name there, weird. Third class – no name there either. What's going on? I can't have done better than that, surely? I move on to second class lower – still no name, am I in the right room? Next is second class upper – and suddenly, there I am. I almost faint again. The next level up from this is a first which as the name suggests, is the highest you can get.

I've done well, I've done really well. I look at the board again just to check it's correct and I'm not, in fact, in the 'Of course you've bloody failed, you droopy pineapple' section. But no, there it is. Wow. I've really passed.

What I didn't do afterwards is celebrate enough. I just headed home, got a summer job counting bras and pants (don't ask) and carried on. When I look back now, I can see that I should have really acknowledged this achievement. Why didn't I hire a lorry, decorate it with my face and dozens of chrysanthemum garlands and parade around the town screaming, 'I DID IT. I BLOODY WELL DID IT!' through one of those loudspeakers.

The thing is, in order to boost and maintain our self-esteem we have to count and celebrate our achievements.

Often our default status is to put ourselves down. 'It's not that big a deal, really.' 'Oh, it was nothing' or 'It was fate more than anything', 'I had a lot of help, it was more of a team effort'. Self-deprecation, the fancy word for not bigging yourself up, is really not good.

I'm not saying you have to celebrate everything, if you start skipping down the street because you opened the fridge door then we may need to talk, but you need to feel pride in what you achieve because it cements the message that you're worthy.

You can also add in a list of the stuff you want to accomplish and then give it a humongous tick when you've done it. That feels sooooo good. I do this with house jobs, I write down on my phone to sweep the leaves in the garden, then once I've done it, I add a tick and boy I love that feeling. I may do a small dance too.

Getting a new job, travelling alone, finishing an art project, scoring a goal at five-a-side, completing a half marathon, baking a killer cake, getting to the top of the climbing wall, successfully navigating a countryside walk, writing a poem, raising money for charity, quitting smoking – whatever it may be. If it felt like hard work and you got there, this is the time for celebration, people.

Get out the floral bunting, put your best disco trousers on and feel great about what you've done and who you are.

71

17. Self-care and not just your hair

I'm living in Edinburgh. I don't know anyone, I've never been to the city before and as I sit in my new flat, I'm thinking 'What the hell am I doing here?'

It's hard to meet new friends because I don't have a job yet or a lot of money to spare. The counselling course I'm doing is part-time and I haven't the courage to ask anyone to go for a drink or a coffee – they seem to have their own lives with families and mates and there's no room for me.

The sun starts to set at three thirty in the afternoon and, like an overdramatic character in a nineteenth-century gothic novel, the darkness seems to match my mood. 'Woe is me. Forsooth, the night is now part of my cursed soul'– that kind of thing.

Am I feeling sorry for myself? You betcha. But the trouble is because I'm feeling so worthless, I stop looking after myself because I think I'm of no value. 'Why should I care for me when I'm not a good person.' I think I may have read this in the same nineteenth-century gothic novel actually.

I start drinking a bottle of wine a night in my tiny bedroom which overlooks the tenement roofs and the large foreboding expanse of The Meadows, the city's big green park. I begin to smoke more cigarettes than normal, at least a pack a day. I stop eating regular meals and just steam a few carrots in the evening. I'm dangerously thin. I don't see anyone. I don't do any exercise. When I reply to a dating advert in the local paper, he doesn't reply, which cements the worthlessness. The bastard, how dare he not want to marry me on the spot.

After a while, I had to look at what I was doing to myself, because things were just circling downwards. Strangely enough, drinking too much, smoking too much, taking no exercise, having no support, having no friends, no meaningful activity and not eating, doesn't do your mind or body any good. Who knew?

I started to look at self-care habits that would build me up not run me down. I started with food. Somewhere I'd heard that you have to eat more than a few carrots a day to survive. Amazing advice. I started having a decent lunch first and, blimey, I actually felt like I had more energy to do stuff. What sorcery was this? Then I moved on to breakfast and discovered I could have energy in the morning too! Gosh. After keeping this up for a while, I finally graduated to

73

a proper meal in the evening. Hurray! Then I cut down the cigarettes I was smoking and lo and behold, I could walk further than before. Eventually I gradually reduced my alcohol intake which improved my mood no end; no more forlorn gazing out of the window. I got a part-time job and the interaction with others gave me motivation to keep going.

Looking after ourselves is crucial to self-esteem because if we don't think we're worthy, we tend to engage in activities that harm us – we assume we're undeserving of the effort. We have to reverse that.

When you continue to harm yourself, it gets harder and harder to see a way out, because you also feel the shame of what you're doing. So, even if you think you're terrible and not worth looking after, I want you to start to take care of yourself. If you can't do it for you, do it for me.

In order to tackle your emotional needs, we have to start with your physical needs. Take a look at what you can do to look after yourself more. How can you get better sleep? How can you eat better? How can you cut down on the things that harm your body? How can you fit in some physical exercise?

You have to invest in yourself so you can see that you're worthy. Every act of self-care cements that we're worthy. Every act of self-harm cements that we're not. Every small action that indicates you're of worth, is a long-term move towards valuing yourself.

You take a walk in a park in springtime and sit under a tree for an hour. You head off to see a concert and boogie at the back of the arena. You make yourself a batch of hearty soup. You play badminton with your best friend once a week. You crochet a blanket for winter nights. You get emotional support through counselling and things start to build and build.

Soon, valuing yourself becomes a habit, it's just what you do: you look after yourself because you think you're of worth.

18. Billy, AKA the Notorious Self-talk Bully

I call the inner critic inside my head, Billy the Notorious Self-talk Bully – but his rap name is just Billy STB.

I've created him to make it easier to see how ridiculous our thoughts are. He's a real knobhead, a complete bullying loser.

I'm going to show you, by the power of role play, just how stupid Billy is and how your thoughts are stupid too. Notice I said your thoughts are stupid, not 'you're stupid'; you're lovely and I really like what you've done with your hair today.

Now, there is nothing quite as dreadful as being on a training course and the instructor going, 'So now, everyone, I'm going to pair you up with someone you intensely dislike and I want one of you to take the role of the parsnip and the other the gardener and we're going to assess your ability to grow. Role play this for forty minutes without stopping, then swap. Afterwards we'll recreate that role play in front of the whole group when it will also be live-streamed to the whole organisation, who will be scoring you out of one hundred and if you go below ninety-eight you'll lose your job. Okay?'

I digress. Here is how the role play with me and Billy went.

BILLY: You're useless.

ME: It's true, I am.

BILLY: You're a bad person.

ME: Yes, you're right.

BILLY: You're a terrible husband.

ME: I can't argue with that.

BILLY: You're lazy.

ME: Yes.

BILLY: You've achieved nothing.

ME: Again, true.

BILLY: You're stupid.

ME: Definitely.

BILLY: You're unlovable.

ME: I am.

BILLY: You're ugly.

ME: Absolutely.

BILLY: No one likes you.

ME: They don't.

BILLY: You can't do anything right.

ME: Nothing at all.

BILLY: You fail at life.

ME: I do.

BILLY: You're rubbish at your job.

ME: Indeed.

BILLY: You don't deserve happiness.

ME: I couldn't agree more.

This is what Billy says to me all the time. The question, therefore, is: why the hell am I listening to such a gaslighting, bullying idiot?

I want you to read it again but out loud this time, taking the role of Billy. Fear not, this is not an exercise in embarrassing you, it has a purpose. You see, the first time I heard it out loud and not just in my head, it really made me realise how utterly ridiculous my self-talk was. It cemented how ludicrous it was and it's really important that we understand that.

Give it a go now. You can absolutely go off to a quiet room or down the bottom of the garden or to a dark park at three o'clock in the morning, should you wish to.

Did you read it out loud? If you didn't and thought, 'I'm not going to blummin' well do that, James will never know', I want you to actually do it.

Did you hear how nonsensical it sounds? Did you listen to yourself as Billy said those stupid words? Hopefully it's enough for you to go, 'Yes, jeez, my inner self-talk bully is a complete flatulent weasel of the highest order, I'm never going to listen to it again, ever. Ever. Ever.' If so, hurrah, have a celebratory mojito.

I do this exercise whenever Billy starts shouting at me. I clock it's Billy talking to me and then say his words out loud and see how ludicrous they really are, because the more ridiculous something is, the less power it has over you.

19. Don't use crutches unless you have a broken leg

We're going to go back about twenty-five years. I'm in my flat in Glasgow with my flatmate Sal. She's worried that I'm smoking too much. Picture her on one side of the sofa and me, chain smoking after a particularly hideous day at work, on the other.

She's right that I'm smoking too much, and I've developed a particularly alluring cough each morning which makes me sound like a cat bringing up a dozen furballs – really sexy. Oh and, just to add to the picture, there's a bottle of red wine on the table and I've drunk most of it. That's become a problem too because when we head to the pub, I need a gazillion drinks to feel even vaguely worthwhile. Okay, I need to confess there is also a large bowl of doughnuts by my side – I've eaten eleven.

Sal is looking at me as I take another slurp of wine and says, 'Is this an act of self-love or self-harm, James?'

'What?' I say, a bit perplexed.

'You heard me,' she says pointing to the table. 'All this: the drinking, the smoking, eating these doughnuts – if you can call them that, they're so hideous – are they acts of self-love or self-harm?'

This stops me in my tracks, and I put down the doughnut that's halfway to my mouth.

'They make me feel better,' I say.

'But are they really helping your self-esteem in the long term?' continues Sal. 'Because, from where I'm sitting, all I can see is you using these things as a crutch because you don't like yourself and, let's be honest, they're not doing a great job.'

81

Bugger. I look at the cheap red wine, the menthol flavoured cigarettes and the pink doughnuts with rainbow sprinkles on them and realise she has a point. A very big point – so big it's stabbing me in the stomach, although that might be my intestines trying to process the doughnuts.

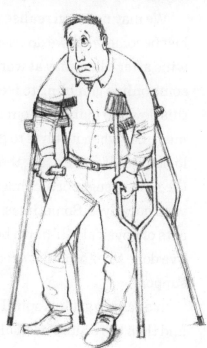

When our self-worth is low, we can start to rely on things to make us feel better in the short term, like alcohol, drugs, smoking, shopping sprees, or crappy food, but these things will never do the heavy lifting to raise our self-esteem in the long term.

If, like me, you're using these things to feel better about yourself, we need to have a talk. A bit like the chat Sal had with me all those years ago.

Now, I'm by no means perfect now. I often buy overpriced high sugar content yoghurts because the packaging tells me it contains 'organic Belizean passionfruit, picked by the freshly moisturised hands of modern-day vestal virgins, gently harvested only on nights the moon is slowly waning'.

We may not even realise we're using crutches, it's just become what we do on a regular basis. A bottle of wine after a busy day at work to feel more like ourselves, some online gambling to feel more 'us'. We might put this down to managing our stress, or some entertainment, but when it starts to get more serious, we have to look to see if we're using them to escape. You see, after the rush of sugar or alcohol or adrenalin, we're still left with ourselves. Sometimes, we may do more serious acts of physical self-harm because we hate ourselves, I've done this too and it's really important to get support.

It's easy to get in a spiral of using crutches to help and then the crutch itself also becomes a problem. For example, we drink to feel better but then the drinking becomes a problem because we can't stop. Then we have two problems, not just one.

We know that rich celebrities can feel as bad about themselves as we mere mortals do. Expensive cars don't make them feel better, diamond-encrusted slippers don't raise their self-esteem – and I am more than happy to test this theory by the way, if someone wants to buy me a superyacht. Relying on things like wealth, status or beauty to raise our self-esteem will only make us feel hollow, which, when you *really* think about it, is not a good thing.

Also, why would anything external work to perman- ently raise your self-esteem? It just doesn't make sense. If someone had discovered the solution to low self-esteem was to eat doughnuts, then we all would have done that – and, boy, did I try.

We always, always, always need to think long term and consider what Sal asked, 'Ultimately, is this an act of self- love or self-harm?' We have to look closely at the things we rely on to feel better about ourselves and if they're not raising our esteem (which they won't), then we need to make changes.

I am here to tell you that the reward for relying on ourselves and loving ourselves is so much better than any doughnut is going to be – including the fudge and choc- olate ones with a sugar glaze.

83

Real self-esteem is built from within you, not on the things you think you need to rely on.

84

20. I like big buts

Warning, this chapter will contain puns on the word bottom. Yes, I am actually seven years old.

I'm in my garden with my friend Noah, observing my attempts to make my outside space look like Monet's garden at Giverny, which isn't easy when it's not a glorious two-and-a-half acre plot on the banks of the River Seine.

Noah just has to look at some seeds and they immediately sprout into a flourishing lemon tree. Me? Well . . . not so much, so I'm having a go at myself.

'I can't get anything to grow,' I say. 'I'm a rubbish gardener.'

'But look at all the amazing things that *are* growing,' says Noah. 'There are gorgeous geraniums, a lovely shrub over there and your camelia is always stunning.'

I look around and realise he's right, things are actually growing. Okay, okay it doesn't look like a miniature Kew Gardens, but it's silly to call myself a rubbish gardener.

After Noah leaves, having taken multiple cuttings

which he will transform into healthy plants and win numerous horticulture awards along the way, I start thinking about what he said and his use of the word 'but'. You see, using 'but' is really important when challenging our self-esteem so I try it out on other negative self-talk.

'I feel unlovable BUT there are people that love me.'

Hmm . . . it does seem to work. I try some more.

'I feel like a failure BUT there are things I've achieved.'

'I feel ugly BUT there are people who find me attractive.'

Interesting how it seems to work, isn't it? If I use the word 'but' and then look at the actual evidence, it reveals the truth of the situation instead of the negativity my self-esteem brain is presenting.

Add the word 'may' into the sentence and it dilutes the bile even more.

'I may feel like a terrible partner BUT that's not what they tell me.'

'I may feel unemployable, BUT I've held down jobs in the past.'

Practise saying this when your negative self-talk is getting loud. You use this sentence structure:

'I may feel like . . . . BUT . . . . '

It starts to undo the nonsense we're telling ourselves because all self-talk loves a certainty. You see, life is grey, not black and white, it's never just one thing or another.

Saying 'I'm a terrible gardener' leaves no room for debate, evidence and reality.

When we have low self-esteem, we never think 'Oh, I'm kind of a terrible person sometimes, maybe just a little bit.' It's always, 'I'm a terrible person.' Full stop. As if the statement isn't up for negotiation. That's what the BUT does; it opens up negotiations, it dilutes the certainty.

I do this whenever a definite negative self-talk pops into my head and it really works. I'll be cooking and put too many dried herbs in the casserole. 'I'm a terrible cook,' my brain says. Then I introduce 'but' and change it to 'I may feel like a terrible cook, but I made a really nice lasagne last week.'

Give it a go. You could start with, 'I may feel like I have a horrible butt, but that's not what the rear of the year competition said about my butt when I came second and was given a "runner up" sash, to go round my butt.' Or you could find a better example, it's entirely up to you.

21. This chapter is sponsored by Elvis

We're going to have a think about how much your self-hating has helped your self-esteem. I want you to head into a garden or park, put your fist under your chin and do an impression of Rodin's sculpture *The Thinker* and start pondering.

I mean, has it actually helped at all?

Has telling yourself that you're an awful person done anything other than make you feel worse? Has berating yourself your whole life been fruitful in any way? I'm guessing not, because it hasn't helped me at all – which is why I've given it up.

Hating yourself leads to more hating of yourself because you get into a weird train of thought in which you start hating yourself even more, because you're hating yourself. Does that makes sense? Sometimes, I realise I'm hating myself and then I'll be so cross that I'm doing it that my self-esteem goes even further down.

It may seem obvious but let's be very, very, very, very, VERY clear:

'Hating yourself is not the solution to your low self-esteem'

Now, this isn't just a case of going, 'Yeah, alright James, whatever, I already know that.' We really need to keep this at the forefront of our minds because it's a way to stop the spiralling of self-hate. By the way, *Spiralling of Self-Hate* is also the name of my one-man thrash metal band, touring in a town near you.

It's a way of interrupting the self-hate process, a kind of stop sign on the low self-esteem highway.

When the self-hating starts, the criticising, the thoughts that you're not good enough, what we do is imagine Elvis holding a big sign saying:

'Hating Yourself is Not the Solution to Your Low Self-esteem'

I'm not quite sure why it's Elvis; I think it's something about the lovely curl of the lip that stops me in my tracks. He also goes 'nah huh' and waves his finger in an Elvisy way. He's smiling as well, which is nice. Know that Elvis loves you and believes in you.

89

Anyone from the Elvis Presley estate, if you want to sponsor this book, that is absolutely fine with me. We can come to some mutually fulfilling arrangement – I am totally willing to accept an eight-bedroom, fifteen-bathroom Beverly Hills mansion as an initial down payment. I'm a reasonable guy after all.

Hate never achieved much when you think about it. Anger might fuel some motivation, but loathing and bitterness never achieves much and it's the same with self-esteem.

Hating is the opposite of what we want to do, so why do we spend so much time doing it to ourselves? Well, because we're trapped in a self-hating loop and Elvis helps us stop that loop with his big sign. Oh yes.

And you know what? When you manage to stop the self-hate, when you realise that all the hating is achieving nothing, then you feel free and released from the hate trap and, if I may say so, that's the wonder, the wonder of you.

22. Name it, frame it, reframe it

Thoughts are tricky blighters, aren't they? They're just thoughts though, not actions. So when I think about punching the person on the train for playing loud German techno music without headphones, it's just a thought; no one has got hurt. Well, not yet anyway.

But low self-esteem thoughts are a bit different because they can weigh us down and lower our self-esteem even further. Especially when things don't go our way.

Recently, I applied for a part-time job. I was quite excited as I thought it sounded really interesting and I'd be doing more work in mental health. I really hoped I stood a chance of an interview so I went ahead and put my application in. I got an interview, which was great, but it coincided with plans I'd made to go to a book festival. Typical. So I had to sit in a car in a supermarket car park and do the video call – not ideal circumstances for a job interview.

I thought I had answered the questions thoroughly and the panel seemed to smile a lot, although this could have been because people kept passing with their weekly groceries, pushing loud shopping trolleys to their cars and shouting 'Jean! Jean! Did you pick up those purple topped turnips? They're two for one this weekend.'

I didn't get the job. There were two posts and I got neither of them. So how to deal with this? Now, obviously I was disappointed. I have work and personal experience in mental health and write a series of mental health books. I certainly didn't think it was a dead cert I would get one of the roles, but I was hopeful because I'd got to the interview stage.

My self-esteem started to plummet. I'm hopeless, I thought to myself, I probably rambled on about yoghurt, told some stupid jokes and called them all by the wrong names. Why did I bother applying when it was all going to be a disaster anyway? I'm unemployable and a complete moron.

This went on for days. Berating myself, feeling crap about each and every part of my life. The self-esteem spiral had started running downhill and I couldn't catch it. By the time the head of panel emailed to ask if I'd like feedback, I was so worn down and tired I just agreed because it was the easiest thing to do.

They said I interviewed well, but other people had given more detailed answers to a few questions and that's why I didn't get the job. Lying on my bed reading the email and mulling things over, I suddenly realised how my negative self-talk had made things so much worse.

This is when I came up with the 'Name it. Frame it. Reframe it' system. Apparently, I have great ideas when I hate myself – who knew? You see, I realised what I needed to do next time was to look at things differently. It goes like this:

93

NAME the thoughts that are going on in your head and tell yourself this is your low self-esteem talking. This helped me to realise that the thoughts had been triggered by not getting the job.

Put a **FRAME** around it, which means you put a box around *just* the thoughts relating to the trigger and don't let them seep into all the other parts of your life. Stop the spiral before it begins. The frame helps me ensure I don't go to more extremes and start hating every part of myself. Starve the thought, don't give it oxygen to grow. Don't pull on the self-esteem thread.

Then **REFRAME** it – which is the most important part. This isn't a case of going, 'Oh well, there are bunnies frolicking in the hills and beautiful flowers in the meadows so everything is fine.' It's not being positive about something that genuinely hurts. But it is being realistic and understanding what's happening. I understood that I hadn't given thorough enough answers to the questions and that was something I could do next time. I also reminded myself that just because I didn't get one job, didn't mean that I was unworthy in all aspects of my life. It's simply that I didn't do well enough this time – that's all. I'm not going to get every job that I apply for. You don't reframe into something sweetly positive, you reframe it into something realistic.

When something negative happens, you use the 'name it, frame it, reframe it' system to get your thinking back in order.

23. Create a confident confidante called Connie

I have multiple imaginary friends. No, I'm not six years old, well at least physically, but I do find made-up mates help me immeasurably.

It's not as whacky as it sounds, trust me. These buddies are the kind of people that you strive to be and have qualities that you want to develop. It's a way of using your imagination to channel the parts of you that you want to change.

No doubt some eminent psychologist called Eric (they're all called Eric) has given this process a name, but I am not an eminent psychologist, so you'll just have to trust me that it works, because it does.

One of the people I create in my head is my old mucker, Connie. Connie is a complete legend. She knows what she's about, she doesn't doubt herself, she trusts her instincts, she's not swayed by what others think, she thinks she's okay. She stands with complete composure, she doesn't shirk from tasks. She's not arrogant. She's not up herself. She just lives her life with assurance and, most of all, confidence.

I used Connie to great effect a few years ago when I was delivering a book talk, which I sometimes do. It was in front of a huge amount of people, like a hugely massive audience. How many people? Jeez, like fifty thousand? One hundred million? I don't know, a lot. Alright, so thinking back it was probably two hundred people, but they were all there looking at me and waiting for me to talk. What was up with that?

I've done talks before; I really like them, especially when people join in and ask questions. But this time, I knew there would be a bigger audience and it was making me panic. Plus, I'd have to wear one of those complicated microphones that you put down your pants, up your shirt and twice around your neck so that you look like a 1940s telephone exchange operator. 'Thank you so much for your call today. Mayfair 351 was it? Just connecting now, madam. Good day to you.'

The more I thought about it, the more I started to panic. What would they think of me? What if my microphone got twisted and my trousers fell down? What if I tripped going onto the stage, was rendered unconscious and then had to be helicoptered out of the building? What if a large, orange dragon attacked me because he hated me and then the audience turned into zombies and came on the stage to collectively bite my ankles? You see, *anything* could happen. *Anything.*

What I needed was a shot of confidence (and possibly a big reality check), so I turned to Connie. I asked myself these questions:

* What would Connie do?
* How would Connie think?
* How would Connie respond?
* How would Connie present herself?
* Can Connie defeat orange dragons?

Now you don't need to fashion an effigy of Connie out of some spare clothes from a charity shop; it's just a case of knowing what Connie would think, imagining her answers and then copying her.

I decided that she would prepare well and practise the speech by recording it on her phone – so I did that. Then I decided that Connie would remember to speak slowly, because when we talk in public we naturally speed up to try and get it over with. Then I decided she would stand as tall as she could and look out at everyone with assurance, knowing they were just other people and not zombies.

Then I decided she would remember to incorporate jokes, because laughing always releases tension in the audience and within yourself. Then I decided she would remember that people wanted to hear me talk; it wasn't as if they had been forced to come in handcuffs from their home screaming, 'No! No! I don't want to go and see that man. Don't make me. I'd rather poke needles into my eyes than go and hear him talk.'

I also decided that she would remember that it was half an hour of my life and that's not a lot of time in the grand scheme of things, so if it didn't quite go to plan, no one will have died, not even of boredom. Then I decided that she would remember that there's a strong possibility that it would be enjoyable, especially as I'd really enjoyed other talks I've done.

And, boy, it really worked.

You can use Connie in lots of situations. She works well for interviews, meeting new people, going on a first date, taking exams, cooking a new meal for friends, arranging a retirement party for a colleague, doing a presentation to the board, joining a badminton class for the first time and preparing to defeat orange dragons. You just need to imagine Connie really well, understand who she is and replicate what she would do.

After a while, the copying becomes part of who you are – it's a kind of 'fake it until you make it' kind of thing. The more you take on these qualities, the more you practise with them, the more they integrate with yourself.

Go forth and get Connie in your life.

24. Don't write a gratitude journal

Okay, I totally lied, I do want you to write a gratitude journal. But we're certainly not calling it a gratitude journal because if I hear one more person going on about how they start their day at 4.30am, do two hours at the gym whilst their goji berry and wheatgrass smoothie is maturing, then head to their meditation room/mindfulness retreat space/sound bath sanctuary in the attic of their twenty thousand square foot summer retreat cabin for five hours of gratitude journaling, with an Egyptian vulture quill and ink from self-sacrificing squids throwing themselves on a Cretan beach, I will absolutely completely explode.

Being thankful is a useful self-esteem tool. Writing stuff down works because it reminds you of the things you already know you're thankful for, but with our busy lives we don't stop to focus on them. Secondly, once we start making a list, we discover new things that make us thankful and bring us joy.

I don't use a journal specifically for my gratitude scribblings – by all means, buy your own, but I was gifted one once and I felt this huge surge of guilt every time I didn't write in it. It sat on my coffee table staring at me all neglected, which just made me feel bad about myself. I became very ungrateful for the gratitude journal.

I have a page on the notes app on my phone and I write my list there. Now, the key is to do a fresh page each day, otherwise you'll do what I did and look at the previous day and go, 'Well, I'm still just thankful for the same stuff.' You will ignore the whole exercise and make some Mexican scrambled eggs or something instead. You can write *some* of the same stuff as you did before, but try and be thankful for something new each day – that's a really important bit.

The other thing that will take a bit of getting used to is the sheer embarrassment of doing it. It feels wrong some-how. It feels weird. It feels a bit boastful. But everything feels weird the first time you do it. Learning to ride a bike felt odd. Same for swimming or baking a cake. New shoes always feel odd. The more you do it, the less weird it will feel.

What I don't do is write down that I'm thankful for something at another's expense. For example, 'I'm so glad I'm tall and not short like some men.' Or, 'I'm so thankful that I'm better looking than the guy down the road.' That's not how this works. Our thankfulness needs to be what's in our *own* lives not in comparison to other people's, otherwise we're using other people's misfortunes to bolster our esteem and that's ineffective and, you know, just not a cool thing to do.

Start off by doing it every day to get some practice. Once you've done it for a few months, you can drop down to every week, like me. It's nice to do this at the end of the week, a kind of summing up of things. Here's an extract from mine. Notice that I use 'thankful for' rather than gratitude, so it won't make me puke.

I'm Thankful For:

* My husband, even though he never changes the toilet roll
* My cats, even though they live in my flat rent free
* My ability to move, to cycle and to get around easily
* My friends, for their love and always making me laugh
* My family for their unwavering support
* The ability to travel and see amazing things
* A flock of starlings I saw at lunchtime flying over the pier
* Some beautiful blue flowers growing wild
* Seeing a fantastic concert last night

Sometimes, I'm halfway through writing the list and a thought pops into my head like, 'I'm not bloody well thankful for my depression and friggin' anxiety', but then I have to stop, take a breath and go back to the things I am thankful for. Otherwise, it can be easy to go down a road of all the things I'm *not* grateful for, which is often an easier list to write with the help of our low self-esteem. But it is not going to help us in the long run.

Oh, and today I'm thankful to you, for reading this book.

25. Would you say that to a friend?

A few years ago . . . Well, maybe ten years ago. Okay, twenty years ago. Alright, fine you've wheedled it out of me, thirty-four years ago, I got my school exam results. They weren't good. I'm not naturally academic; I can't just rock up to an exam and ace it, I have to do a lot of work just to scrape through.

I'm sat in my bedroom with my piece of paper showing my results and I'm giving myself a really hard time. C for Biology? Really? I thought it was the one science I was good at. D for Maths and an E for Art? Blimey. C for French? *Zut alors!* And after all those extra lessons. Not good, really not good.

Of course, part of the problem with French was that I could only remember the phrase '*Zut alors!*' and so repeated it a lot during my oral exam.

'What sandwiches do you like?' asked the examiner.

'Les, I mean des, I mean umm . . . sandwiches? Errr . . . zut alors! Fromage?'

'Do you like to go swimming?'

'Oui. Zut alors! Je swim a lot dans le sea.'

'Do you have any pets at home?'

'Zut alors! Une cat. Il s'appelle ... zut alors!'

I should have worked harder, I should have been given a better brain, I should have bribed the French examiner with my artwork – no, wait, that probably wouldn't have worked given my recent exam results. I'm giving myself a really hard time.

My friend Simon comes over and we go for a walk to the beach. On the way there I continue to berate myself for my pathetic results. I'm a useless thicko, a deplorable idiot, a shameful mess.

We get to the sea, and I find a few stones to skim into the water and Simon joins me. With each stone that fails to hop across the water, I swear at myself. I can't even skim a stone. I try and hide my tears and wipe them away with the sleeve of my t-shirt.

'Listen,' says Simon. 'All those things you're saying to yourself, I want you to say them to me.'

'What?' I reply. 'I'm not going to do that.'

'Go on, tell me how useless I am, how stupid I am, how I'll never amount to anything. Go on,' says Simon encouraging me.

'No. I won't,' I say.

'You can do it,' says Simon. 'Tell me that I'm worthless,

tell me I never work hard enough.'

'Simon, I can't.'

'Of course you can't,' he replies, 'because that would be ridiculously cruel. So why are you happy to say them to yourself?'

I stop trying to skim the stones and sit down by the water's edge. Simon sits down too and puts an arm around me.

'Why are you treating yourself so much worse than you would a friend?' he asks.

I think for a while. I'm only doing that because I hate myself. There's no other reason. I wouldn't say those words to him or anyone else. What Simon said has really hit home and, to be honest, still hits home all these years later.

You see, it's fine to want to improve and do better, that's great. What's not okay is to treat yourself so badly and I really learned that lesson on the beach. When you start being hard on yourself, I want you to think, 'Would I say that to a friend?' And if you wouldn't then please stop saying it to yourself.

26. Flick the pixie

My friend Helena and I are sat in her house having coffee. I've been having a bad day and am being comforted by her greyhound Madam Fluffkins (it's a long story) who is sat on my lap, occasionally groaning, then silently farting with satisfaction. Let's just say, I'm not entirely happy with Madam Fluffkins farting on me.

> ME: Umm . . . Helena, do you think she's comfortable on my lap?
>
> HELENA: What? Yes, of course, she loves you.
>
> *[fart]*
>
> ME: Right. Excellent. She loves her dog bed too though, doesn't she?
>
> HELENA: Oh, she does. Spends all night in it. Do you want a biscuit?
>
> ME: No, no I couldn't possibly.
>
> HELENA: No probs, I'll put them away.

ME: Okay, sure. Does err . . . I mean, do you think she wants to go onto her bed instead?

HELENA: No, she seems very comfortable on you.

[fart, fart]

ME: Well, that's excellent.

HELENA: She doesn't sit on everyone, she must really like you.

ME: Yes, she must, what an honour.

[fart]

HELENA: But if she's too heavy, I can take her off?

ME: Take her off? No, no, no need for that. It's absolutely fine.

HELENA: Great.

ME: Super.

HELENA: Splendid.

ME: Lovely.

HELENA: James, when are you actually going to tell me you don't want her farting on you?

ME: Farting? Oh no, I don't mind at all. In fact, I wish she would fart more. I'm loving it. How can we make her pass *more* gas?

HELENA: James, please.

ME: Fine, fine, I don't want her farting on me. I've said it, I'm sorry but I just don't find it relaxing.

HELENA: If I hadn't mentioned it, when would you have told me you weren't happy?

ME: I'm sure I would have done. Yes, really quite soon.

HELENA: For goodness' sake, you have to learn to say what you need.

ME: I will. Sorry.

HELENA: And you do want a biscuit, don't you?

ME: Yes, please, I'd like five and one for later.

HELENA: Bit rude of you.

Low self-esteem stops us from speaking up. We don't say what we need, because we think we're not worthy. The world feels too unsafe to be ourselves.

I do this all the time. I don't tell people I'm unwell and ask them to come and look after me. I don't ask people for a hug because I've had a bad week at work. I don't call a friend for a chat as my mental health has got worse. I worry that if I ask for what I need people will think I'm rude and then they'll hate me.

I realised that to tackle my low self-esteem I had to start speaking up, telling people what I needed and not shying away.

Don't get me wrong, I've not been phoning up friends and going, 'Oi, Sarah! Come round 'ere now and attend to my needs.' That sounds a bit rude actually, but you get my drift. It's just that when I need something I don't shrink away and think I'm not worthy enough to ask for things.

I ask if people can look after my cats when I go away. I ask if someone can help me prune the tree in my garden. I ask someone to get some shopping when I've broken my ankle. I ask for support when I'm grieving.

Now, when I do this, a little bugger of a pixie appears resting on my shoulder saying in a high-pitched voice, 'Don't say that! You can't ask them that, you fool, they'll hate you.' What I then do is flick the pixie off my shoulder.

109

Admittedly, it looks a bit weird whilst I'm on the bus flicking my shoulder, but it helps me to remember not to let my low self-esteem get in the way of saying what I need.

The first few times I asked for what I needed it did feel a bit odd, but that's just because I wasn't used to doing it. Now it feels fine. It feels good. I feel empowered, I feel so much better about myself and a little bit like a self-esteem superhero to be honest. I'm quite inclined to get a red cape and some tights.

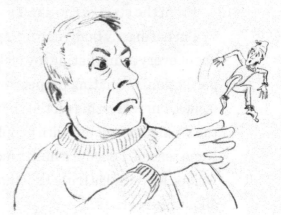

27. Get some perspective

I'm walking in the Welsh countryside with my friend Chloe. I've brought some sandwiches which are slowly congealing together in the bottom of my rucksack and my water bottle is swinging precariously from a strap on the bag.

We trek for about an hour. Well, Chloe treks as she's the true rambler; I trudge along, realising that my boots are not in fact waterproof. I start to complain about this but, as Chloe rightly says, you shouldn't buy outdoor gear from a dodgy car boot sale.

From the start of the day, I've been hating myself.

I'm hating my body, hating my stupid brain that worries about everything, hating my lack of courage, hating my perfectionism, hating my pessimism, hating my anger issues. I'm regretting all the chances I never took, all the stupid arguments with people I've ever had and, for some reason, I devote a huge amount of time to hating my wrists. My mind is truly ridiculous – I mean, who worries about their wrists?

After walking for a couple of hours we take lunch sitting on a rock that looks out to a valley below us. Whilst I eat the congealed sandwiches I've made, I berate myself for not putting them in a container that would stop them becoming one giant cheese and marmite mush. I look at my ridiculous boots that are still letting in the dew from the grass and I think about all the other stupid decisions I've made.

And on and on and on. All day I do this.

I don't notice the beautiful hills curving over the horizon like a partially risen Victoria sponge. I don't see the companionable groups of trees huddling together in a distant field. I don't take in the sun soothing the edges of the dark clouds to the west.

And on and on and on.

I don't see the lambs playing in the field. I don't see the buzzard silently surveying the undergrowth. I don't see the wild orchids hiding under a bush like a birthday surprise.

And on and on and on.

I don't hear my friend telling me about her week. I don't hear her gush about her new lovely girlfriend. I don't hear how she's finally mastered a Thai green curry with the right amount of lemongrass.

I'm a loser, an ugly shrimp head, a weak idiot who should have never been born, a pathetic whinger, a thick piece of slimy mud, an idiotic subhuman.

Now looking back at that day, I see what a complete and utter waste it was.

All I managed to do was to feed my self-loathing. I think of all the happiness I didn't experience, the connection with my friend that wasn't there, all the beauty I didn't see.

Now, this is going to sound a bit grim but bear with me: in a few generations' time, you'll be forgotten. Aren't I the ray of sunshine today, eh? But it's true. Your great-great-grandparents you may have heard about, but you won't have met them, they weren't a part of your life and you probably don't know their names off the top of your head. It will be the same for you.

What I'm getting at here is that life is short, really blummin' short, so it's just not worth spending your time hating yourself.

There are lots of things to be worried about, world news, terrorism, inflation, and then all the day-to-day stuff – what is the gungy stuff coming out of the guinea pig's eye? Who's eaten all the cereal again? Why is the car making that weird throaty sound when you reverse? What we shouldn't do is waste our very precious time feeling rubbish about ourselves.

I often think about the saying, 'Somewhere in the world there is someone who wants what you have.' Generally, I don't like hokey sayings that you could put in a Hallmark card, or inscribe on a piece of bleached driftwood and hang up in the kitchen, but this one does help me. People in a distant country are desperate to live somewhere with sanitation, a roof, with access to clean water, or in a relationship, or any number of things that I currently have.

When we take a wider view on life it really gives us some perspective on our self-esteem issues. There are loads of important things to do. We can find meaning in our careers, build relationships, nurture friendships, love one another – but hating yourself is not one of them.

113

28. You havin' a laugh?

I'm in Bangkok in a beautiful Buddhist temple, with
my amazing Australian guide Tim. He's been living in
Thailand for thirty years, he's married to a Thai woman
and really knows the history of this country. We're here to
see an enormous gold Buddha.

TIM: This is a very special Buddha for the Thai people.

ME: It's really stunning.

TIM: It's fascinating because for many years before it
came here, it was covered in semen.

ME: I'm sorry?

TIM: Yes, it was covered in it.

ME: Covered in it?

TIM: Unusual, eh?

ME: Gosh. That's . . . really, really unusual, Tim.

TIM: Yes.

ME: Incredible. Umm . . . are you sure?

TIM: Am I sure? Yes. There are records of it and photos.

ME: Photos?

TIM: Yes.

ME: Umm . . . why was it covered in it?

TIM: No one really knows, but it took some time to take it off.

ME: I'm sure.

TIM: It makes it very special.

ME: I'll say.

TIM: It took many people to rub it off.

ME: Right. Yes. Absolutely.

TIM: They needed gloves.

ME: Of course.

TIM: Health and safety first.

ME: Gosh, yes.

TIM: But now it's all beautiful again. Take some time to have a proper look and we'll meet back in half an hour.

I walk around the statue and think, that's a heck of a lot of semen to cover a five-tonne Buddha. But I remind myself I

115

mustn't judge other cultures. There are traditional practices that might seem strange to the western eye, but that's what travel is all about, broadening the horizons, experiencing different ways of life, understanding cultures and practices different to my own.

I collect my shoes from outside the temple, which have been nicely guarded by a stray cat, and in the car on the way back to the hotel I ask Tim about the Buddha again, because I really want to understand this semen thing.

ME: So, errr . . . the Buddha.

TIM: Yes. Did you like it?

ME: I loved it.

TIM: It's special, eh?

ME: Yes. Ummm . . . I was just wondering . . .

TIM: Yes?

ME: Well . . . how much – well . . . I mean, it must have taken an awful lot of semen to cover the Buddha.

TIM: What?

ME: Was it some kind of fertility ritual in the countryside?

TIM: No, no . . .

ME: Did they bring the semen from a nearby village that celebrated mutual copulation and fecundity?

TIM: No, no, you've misunderstood.

ME: Is there a record of the actual semen ceremony?

TIM: No. No.

ME: I suppose it was a long time ago.

TIM: No, James. Listen—

ME: You see, I'm fascinated by cultural anthropology, I studied a bit of it in college. You've heard of Margaret Mead, I expect? Probably the leader in her field at the time and of course you can't dismiss Franz Boas, who's often called the father of cultural anthropology, or Daddy B as I call him. Then there's Ruth Benedict, I like her work too—

117

TIM: James.

ME: I wonder if the other statues in the city have a similar history? Were they covered in semen as well? Did that ceremony extend to other Buddhas? Do we know anything about the men that donated? Did they get special recognition from the Dalai Lama?

TIM: That's Tibetan Buddhism and no, James.

ME: No?

TIM: It was cement.

ME: I'm sorry?

TIM: The Buddha, it was covered in cement, not semen.

ME: Cement?

TIM: Yes.

ME: Not semen?

TIM: No.

ME: Cement?

TIM: Yes.

ME: Oh. But you said semen.

TIM: I said cement.

ME: Right, okay. Definitely cement?

TIM: Yes. Definitely.

ME: It wasn't covered in semen?

TIM: Again, no.

ME: I've had a cold and I think I misheard you.

TIM: I think you might have done.

ME: Cement does make more sense now I think about it. My hearing has been bad, yesterday I asked a woman I met about her job as a vet.

TIM: Well, there's nothing wrong with that, is there?

ME: Oh, I know, but it turned out she wasn't saying she was a vet, she was saying that her name was Yvette. She got very confused when I started asking her to diagnose my cat's throaty cough.

Of course, the person who looks a complete and utter dufus in all of this is me, but then we start laughing and don't stop for several minutes. There's nothing like a good belly laugh for the soul.

This incident also helps me to remember to laugh at myself. To take life less seriously. Then we take other people's comments less seriously, then we're not so bothered by the idiot who thinks we'll never amount to anything – when we can laugh them off, we become stronger, we become who we are, a wondrous, fallible being.

When you think about it, we are all ridiculous and there is a freedom to not caring as much. When we try and develop a 'sod it' attitude to life, when we're more carefree, we spend less time thinking about what terrible people we are.

29. Avoid acrimonious alacritous admonishments

I'm heading out to work. I put my socks on, I get the left one on and discover it has a hole in it, 'For goodness' sake James,' I say out loud. 'Why haven't you thrown these out?' I get my jacket from the coat rack and manage to put my arm in the wrong hole, 'Bloody hell, you absolute numpty.' I leave the house and head to the train station and after crossing the road I nearly trip over a small dog who's decided to sniff my ankles. 'James, look where you're going, honestly.' I get to the train station and realise I've forgotten my phone with my ticket on it. 'You complete and utter idiot,' I tell myself and sit down on the bench by the ticket office and rummage in my bag and eventually find it. 'Focus, you fool,' I say. In the meantime, my train has left. 'You pathetic numbskull, now you'll be late for work.'

In the space of ten minutes, I've berated myself five times.

It's so easy to do this – it happens almost without us thinking. Yet, each time we do, our self-esteem takes a battering. These little slips of negative self-talk build up and are just as damaging as the nasty big stuff we say to ourselves.

We wouldn't slap ourselves around the face five times and yet we're happy to inflict five emotional blows without even thinking. These emotional blows are just as bad –and I would argue even worse – than physical blows, because they happen so often, so automatically.

121

What we're going to do is replace the 'oh you idiot' self-talk with kinder words. It takes a bit of effort but it's really important to do. It doesn't matter if you slip up and say the negative stuff; what matters more is that you catch it and change it.

Let's go back to my day trying to get to work and start again, this time saying some nicer stuff to myself.

I'm heading out to work. I put my socks on, I get the left one on and discover it has a hole in it, 'For goodness' sake, James,' I say out loud and *then I stop myself* and say, 'You just forgot to throw them out, do that now and get some more socks.' I get my jacket from the coat rack and manage to put my arm in the wrong hole, 'Bloody hell, you absolute numpty,' *and then I stop myself* and say, 'Easy mistake to make when you're rushing.' I leave the house and head to the train station and after crossing the road I nearly trip over a small dog who's decided to sniff my ankles. 'James, look where you're going, honestly' and *then I stop myself* and say, 'It's easy not to see a small dog. Never mind, no harm done.' I get to the train station and realise I've forgotten my phone with my ticket on it. 'You complete and utter idiot,' I say and *then I stop myself* and say, 'It's probably at the bottom of your bag, take a look.' I sit down on the bench by the ticket office and rummage in my bag. 'Focus, you fool,' I say and *then I stop myself* and say, 'Keep searching calmly.' In the meantime, my train has left. 'You pathetic numbskull, now you'll be late for work,' *and then I stop myself* and say, 'There will be another train along soon, let work know and wait for the next one.'

Do you see what I did? I was just much nicer when I spoke to myself. I was gentler, I was kinder and all this builds up to me appreciating myself more, realising that I'm human like everyone else and not feeding my low self-esteem.

The thing is we all spend *way* too much time giving ourselves a hard time, even about small stuff. 'Damn and blast, I should have known not to step on that rattlesnake that was shaking its tail.' This pushes down our self-esteem really badly. Each time we tell ourselves we should have done better, been better, worked harder, our self-esteem plummets because we're saying we weren't good enough.

Once we start the habit of being hard on ourselves it's tough to stop it and the more we do it the more we believe it. Being constantly hard on ourselves serves no good purpose at all.

So, start catching those admonishments, those automatic harsh words, catch them and then change them and it will start to make a huge difference.

123

30. Get feedback from the people that love ya

I'm currently sat in some uncomfortable underwear. I don't know what's happened, but the waistband has sort of turned over and whenever I try to flip it back it seems to turn over somewhere else and I'm back to square one.

I don't like being uncomfortable. I have a low tolerance for it. I once had to wear some really itchy trousers for school. I hated these trousers. They were the worst trousers in the world. Then I got knocked over in the playground, fractured my skull and ended up in hospital. My first words to my distressed mother were, 'Do I *have* to wear those itchy trousers?' As you can imagine, seeing her son with a massive gash on his head and surrounded by bleeping machines, she agreed I could go for a more comfortable pair. I am a genius, an evil genius but a genius, nevertheless.

Anyway, sometimes we need to get uncomfortable and I'm going to ask you to do something out of your comfort zone. Fear not, I've done this myself so I'm not asking you to try anything I haven't. I want you to get some feedback from your friends that love you. By the way, you can only really do this with your friends; it's way too complicated to do this with family members.

We often make assumptions about those in our lives. Maybe they secretly hate us? Maybe they don't love us at all? Are they only friends with us because we can bake a mean batch of millionaire shortbread? Who knows?

I did this with my friend Leo.

125

ME: I want you to give me some feedback about me.

LEO: *[instantly]* You're a buffoon.

ME: No, listen, I want you to really think about me and then give me some serious feedback.

LEO: You're a big buffoon.

ME: No, really, I want to know how you feel about me. You see, I'm working on my self-esteem and I think it will help to ask the friends what they love about me.

LEO: Okay. Right, I'll think.

[A few seconds pass]

You're still a buffoon.

ME: For goodness' sake.

LEO: Fine, fine. If it's really that important to you.

ME: It is.

LEO: You know we all love you.

ME: But what is it that makes me lovable?

LEO: Blimey, Mr Needy. Okay, you really want to do this?

ME: Yes, I really do.

LEO: Because you're kind.

ME: Right. Anything else?

LEO: You want more?

ME: If there is any.

LEO: I'll have to think again. It may take some considerable time.

ME: Oh, bugger off.

LEO: Okay, okay. You're funny and a good listener and compassionate and supportive and passionate and, well, you're just James. I love you for your bravery and being a good mate and always having my back.

ME: Thank you. That wasn't so difficult, was it?

LEO: Well, the main reason I love you is of course that you make great millionaire shortbread, but I felt I had to come up with some other reasons too.

Unless we ask people for feedback, we never really know what they think about us and, more importantly, when we ask and they give us positive feedback it nourishes our self-esteem. I trust you have more willing friends than my mate Leo. You can say you're reading a book about self-esteem and I've asked you to do it if it makes it easier.

After you've spoken to your mates, write down what they've said and then I want you to compare it to what you say about yourself. Here's a quick comparison I did.

Stuff I say about myself	Stuff my friends said about me
I'm useless	We're so proud of your achievements
I'm a bad person	You're really kind
I hate how I look	We love you for you, not how you look
I'm weak	You're so strong
I can't bake anything	You make great millionaire shortbread
I'm unlovable	We love you

Once you start comparing the two you really have to see that the thoughts about yourself are utter nonsense.

31. Captain fun times

I'm alone on a tree swing in a village, way out into the country. Some kindly person has rigged it up opposite the church and wild flowers are growing around the bank. It's an idyllic scene.

It's been a while since I've been on any kind of swing and this one looks quite complicated to get on. I try to stop it spinning and then attempt to quickly hoist one leg over the wooden seat, but as soon as I do it gets away from me and I hop around for a few seconds trying not to fall on the ground. As someone passes, I try and style it out by skipping around and looking at the flowers, as if this is a completely normal thing for a person to do. They wave their walking stick and smile knowingly, obviously used to seeing people do this kind of contortionist act.

Eventually, after about ten minutes, in a kind of kung-fu like lunge, I manage to wrestle both legs over and grab the rope for dear life as it whooshes out. I kick out from the bank and freewheel into the air as the rope twists and spins me around.

This is wonderful.

Really wonderful.

I feel like a child, carefree, happy. What I wasn't expecting was to feel so great about myself, but I do. I'm happy and content and know that I'm okay. It's weird that a tree swing can help my self-esteem and my confidence, but it has.

Of course, it's not the tree swing itself that is improving my self-worth, although wouldn't it be completely magical if that was the answer? It's the fact that I'm having fun. And it's not just all the dopamine and serotonin whooshing around my brain; it's because fun is fabulously indulgent – a supreme act of self-worth.

You see, when we feel we have no value, we also feel that we shouldn't be having fun. There should be no enjoyment in our lives because we're not worthy of it. So, we don't go and play on the tree swing, we don't go rollerblading on the seafront, we don't hire a rowing boat at the park, we don't sledge down the snowy hill.

We encourage children to have fun all the time. It helps them learn, but also feel good about themselves and that's a brilliant thing. Fun should not be limited to children, adults need it too. We're saying to ourselves that we're worthy of happiness and joy, simply put:

Fun fuels self-esteem.

129

Now, you may think, 'Excellent, with James's permission I can go and get lathered on German sparkling wine for the evening and then dance round the sitting room in just a pair of sparkly tights.' Well, yes and no. By all means, enjoy a tipple – I do too – but I'd like you to try the dancing around the sitting room in just a pair of sparkly tights without copious amounts of alcohol in your system. Mainly because I want you to remember your fun, not block it out with flavoured ethanol, as nice as it can be. You can wear sequin tights rather than sparkly tights, so don't accuse me of not giving you options.

The way I see it, life is about love and it's about moments of joy. Increase your fun and joy and you start to appreciate yourself and like yourself so much more.

32. Moral codes

I'm at university in America and I've been asked to run a
stall showing fellow students what life is like in the UK.
I've got mince pies, a picture of fish and chips and a photo
of a pub with a red phone box outside it. It's not the most
fantastic display, but I've made a commitment and I've
only got to be there for a few hours.

It's part of a day celebrating diversity, something I'm
passionate about. Some people say hello, take a union
jack flag and I fend off questions about rain – yes, it does
rain rather a lot. Big Ben? No, that's the name of the bell,
actually. The royal family – we're not actually related, no.
It's all going okay. Everyone, without fail, says 'cheerio' in a
bad Mary Poppins-esque British accent when they leave.

A friend then comes by and tells me he and others are
off to the woods to pass the afternoon drinking. I explain
I've got to be here for a couple more hours, but he says
everyone is going and I don't really need to stay, there are
plenty of other stalls.

Most of me knows I've made a commitment and wants to help. The other bit of me is worried about being left out. What if everyone has fun without me? 'Come on, James,' he says. 'It won't be the same without you.' So, I pack up quickly and make a run for it, just as the organiser starts to come over with a worried expression to ask me where I'm going.

All afternoon as my friends sit by the waterfall and drink beer, I feel terrible. Really terrible. I don't enjoy myself, I don't laugh, I don't drink any beer. I've let myself down badly and now I hate myself.

I've gone against my own moral code.

When I've made a commitment to do something, whenever possible, I do it, unless I've lost my spleen in a kayaking accident or something. I do my best not to let people down who are relying on me. I'm polite and don't just rush off unannounced to drink beer in the woods. And finally, of course, I've let king and country down and should be hung, drawn and quartered in the Tower of London, the remains of my pathetic body pecked by starving ravens.

We all have a moral code that forms who we are, what we stand for and what we think is important. This comes from our upbringing, from our peers and from the perceptions we form in our minds of the world. We always know when we've gone against it because it doesn't feel good.

When we stick to our guns, we feel much better about ourselves.

I was once on a train with my husband Patrick, heading back home after going to the theatre. A gang of men drinking lager got on. They were shouting and singing a football song. Don't ask me what team they were supporting or what the song was or what match they had been to see, I honestly have no idea. One of them, a particular giant of a man, sat opposite me and next to Patrick. 'So, where have you two been then?' he asked. Slightly anxious, I told him we'd been to the theatre. 'Theatre? Bloody hell. I didn't realise people still went to the theatre.' He goes on to tell us that he's just back from a football match and they lost so he's drowning his sorrows. We chat about football for a bit, but this is a fairly limited conversation topic, as all I know is that at the top of the division people get paid about four million pounds an hour and live in very glitzy houses. My husband knows even less.

Apparently, he can't go abroad to watch England games anymore because he's been banned for fighting and at the moment the government have taken his passport off him. I laugh and then realise he's not joking. And then gulp rather loudly.

Now, I'm really, really, really trying not to judge the fact that he's clearly a very violent man, because to have your passport removed sounds kind of serious to me. I'm also trying (and failing) not to feel afraid of this six-foot-eight giant of a man created entirely out of muscle and Heineken. 'So . . .' he says drinking from his can, 'you guys a couple or what?'

Seconds seem to tick past, slower than a dodgy VAR replay – ooh, hello, maybe I do know about football – and I think should I tell him the truth and risk getting my teeth knocked out, or should I just lie, lie, lie, pretending we are just a couple of good mates and, yes, we do love a lager after the match too.

My husband starts to mumble but doesn't come out with any coherent words. I think, 'I can be true to myself, or I can deny myself,' so I say, 'Yes, we are.' He instantly slaps me hard on the arm and says affectionately, 'That's great that, I love the gays, so does my missus,' and then he smiles broadly and gets off at his stop with his friends, still drinking and singing.

We look at each other somewhat stunned. I've never, ever, been hit so hard in my life, the bruise lasts for weeks, goodness knows what it would be like to be hit by him in anger.

As well as being fantastic proof of times changing and increased tolerance (at least to gay men, possibly less so if you're a football supporter from the opposing team), it was a clear example of being proud to have been myself. I didn't suddenly fake a rough voice and go, 'Oi, well guv, no we're not a bleedin' couple, we're the best of mates who just happen to like to attend musical theatre matinees.' I said it proud. I said it loud – well loud-ish. I came away feeling great about myself because I was true to who I am. I kept to my moral code of never denying being gay, never lying about my marriage.

When we act within our own moral code, we feel proud of ourselves and maintaining this is essential to our self-esteem. For example, if someone is trying to persuade you to run away from a restaurant without paying but instead you stick to your core belief (see Chapter 14) that this is wrong, you will feel much better about yourself for it.

135

33. Telling Billy to bugger off

We have to get angry. Really angry. We have to rage against the negative self-talk because otherwise it will come and eat us up.

Anger is a powerful force. It can do horrendous things, but it can be hugely beneficial when we use it in the right way. Lots of change is fuelled by anger – the women's suffrage movement, the civil rights movement, any battle for equality has anger and injustice at its heart and we're going to harness those feelings.

We're not getting angry with ourselves, you understand. Frankly, there's enough of that already. What we're going to do is turn our low self-esteem thoughts into a person. If you've read Chapter 18, you'll know I call this person Billy. Bloody Billy. We get angry with the *thought* not with ourselves.

Why should you be at the mercy of your low self-esteem? Why should you have to listen to those voices in your head? Bugger all that to hell and back. We should feel angry about low self-esteem taking over our lives.

When we hear Billy's voice in our head going . . .

'You're repulsive.'

'You're worthless.'

'You're useless.'

. . . we fight back.

Now, you can't physically hit your inner voice, clearly, but we can still tell it to bugger off. Loudly. Really bloody loudly. All bullies need to be stood up to and then they start to shrink. Billy is no different.

This is what I do all the time. A thought comes into my mind – and bear in mind it is just a thought, it's not a real thing – and I tell it where to go. The conversation goes like this.

'You're repulsive.'

'Bugger off.'

'You're worthless.'

'Bugger off.'

'You're useless.'

'Bugger off.'

See how easy it is? And the more you do it, the more you get angry and cross and stroppy and annoyed and irate and indignant, the more you're cementing that the voice is wrong.

The more we do stuff in our conscious brain, the more

it seeps into our unconscious brain. Eventually we believe it automatically without thinking. Soon, we start to recognise the negative self-talk as just talk, not the truth, just lies and bluster and nonsense that needs calling out.

Our anger is a conscious act that says we won't put up with the negative self-esteem thoughts going around in our heads. We're saying we're better than some stupid thought. Retaliating pushes the thought back. Answering back bolsters our confidence and raises up our self-esteem.

Bugger off, bugger off, bugger off.

Shout it, scream it, get angry.

34. What are you looking at?

I want to tell you about a walk I went on. It was to try and 139
find perfect people with perfect bodies.

I went up the pedestrianised street near my house,
which has charity shops, coffee shops and those cool shops
that just seem to sell soap, ceramic vases and overpriced
arty scarfs. I had a look for perfect people. I looked all over.
To the point where people were getting suspicious of the
bald, speccy guy gazing at them. I really couldn't find any.
I went into the bookshop, I went into the ironmongers, I
got an Earl Grey tea and a scone in a nice new tea shop and
looked – nada, nothing, nicht, no perfect people.

Now, clearly beauty is in the eye of the beholder,
but there was nobody I could find that matched per-
fection. Funny that? Maybe it's because NO ONE IS
BLOODY PERFECT AND WHAT DOES PERFECT
MEAN ANYWAY AND WHY THE HELL ARE WE SO
OBSESSED WITH HOW PEOPLE LOOK?

That's me shouting by the way.

It's sheer stupidity for our self-worth to be tied up with our appearance. What are we saying here, that if I don't look like a ravishing twenty-one-year-old model that I'm not a worthy human being? That's clearly nonsense.

And what I think is the 'perfect' person, someone else would disagree with so it's all relative anyway. The old adage is 'look good, feel good', when in fact it should be 'look however you want and still feel bloody good', but I guess that's not such a catchy soundbite.

Why would it work that if you look slightly different from 'the norm' – whatever the hell that is – that you're less of a person? Think about it for a moment. That makes absolutely no sense. Most of our low self-esteem thoughts don't make any sense.

We need to divorce our physical appearance from our self-worth. It's not just trial separation time here, it's full-on divorce court, it's over, divide up the vinyl, separate the bank accounts and move on. It's a load of poo trash.

We need to work towards a middle ground with how we view our appearance, not 'I am a demi goddess of ethereal beautification', nor 'I am so ugly I detest each and every particle of my body', just 'I'm okay with my body'.

Our bodies are simply the shell that we live in. You don't hear about crabs hating their bodies, do you? There aren't lobsters going, 'If only my claws were bluer, then I would really love myself.' Crayfish aren't grumbling about the extra few pounds they've put on over the holidays. I don't know why I've gone off on a crustacean-based metaphor, but I'm sure you get my meaning.

The more we worry about our body not being 'perfect', the more time we waste not living our lives. Spending our whole time going, 'If my nose was thinner, if my chin was more defined, if my stomach was flatter, then I would love myself,' is ridiculous. Let me tell you, I've been down this road and correcting these things doesn't make you love yourself, because you just find another part of your body to hate.

141

It's a body and, yes, we should look after it, but that's all it is: a vessel. It's not the essence of us. Say it again: your body is not the essence of you. And again: your body is not the essence of you. One more time: your body is not the essence of you.

You are valid and gorgeous and worthy no matter what you look like and if you start doubting this, I want you to imagine me looking at you in a supportive but also very disapproving way, giving you a hard stare.

Here endeth the lesson.

35. Stop people pleasing, but please love me

I'm at a party I really don't want to be at, but I promised an acquaintance I'd attend and I've run out of viable excuses.

'Very unfortunately, I have to attend my hamster's parents evening.'

'My deceased Great Aunt is giving her first live poetry recital that evening, I'm afraid.'

'Sadly, I've agreed to singlehandedly windsurf around Cape Dubouzet that night. What's that? Where is it? It's ... well, it's in Antarctica.'

I want to make everyone happy, which is a lot of people to please. It's basically impossible. Because I don't have the ability to say, 'Thank you so much for the invitation but I don't want to come to your party.' I'm now chatting to a group of people who introduce themselves as 'Freelance Digital Alchemists' and all I can think of replying to this is 'Soooo ... is that ummm ... is that ... a nine-to-five role?'

What I want to say is, 'That's not a bloody job title, you

pretentious cock parrots.' But of course, I don't because I want them to love me, so I keep chatting, asking them about what it's like to be based in Antigua 'for most of the year' and sympathise with the poor quality of the public Wi-Fi on the island's western beaches.

I'm exhausted. The person who invited me hasn't even seen me. Everyone is chugging shots of Albanian retsina, shouting loudly when they do, and if I hear one more idiot telling me that 'no one reads books anymore', I shall dismember them limb by limb and feed them to the tarantula in the tank who's looking as pissed off as I am.

I do this all the time, put others' needs before my own. I agree to babysit someone's long-tailed chinchilla for six months. Or when I receive an automatic email asking me to review a product, I spend half a day drafting something and make sure a copyeditor checks it for grammar and sentence structure before submitting. If I don't leave a review, I feel guilty and wonder if the computer now hates me.

When we constantly try to please other people at our own expense, when we want to be loved by everyone, all that happens is that our self-esteem plummets because we ignore our own needs. We're basically saying to ourselves that other people are more important than us.

Clearly, I'm not saying don't go to your grandmother's funeral because you'd rather go trampolining. Just because you don't feel like going to work, I wouldn't recommend emailing them to say you've taken a last-minute flight to Ibiza because 'it has a better vibe than the office'. That's not what this is about.

It's about recognising when you're putting others before yourself and then doing something about it. The more you do this the more you're saying, 'I'm important'. Not 'I'm more important than everyone else', just, 'I'm important, my needs matter'. If you want you can add, 'I promise not to be an arsehole about it.'

Now, there is a massive and very important distinction between being selfish and thinking about yourself. Selfishness is only considering you at the expense of others. This is a crappy thing to be.

Thinking about yourself includes considering others and, crucially, puts you in the picture because **YOU ARE IMPORTANT TOO**. Can you see how I've put that in bold, which means it's really essential?

Questions to ask yourself when situations arise:

* Do I need to do this?
* Am I putting others before myself?
* What are my needs in this situation?
* Am I being an arsehole?
* Am I a freelance digital alchemist?

We shouldn't be at the mercy of others so much that our

self-esteem is impacted. Each decision you make to pri-oritise you is a win for your self-esteem. It's not realistic to get to the point where you don't care at all what people think, we all value affirmation and love from others, but trying is everything.

I took one last look around the party. People were now attacking the buffet with all the grace of a half-starved piranha. Some people were smoking on the balcony and putting the finished butts in the geraniums. I waved good-bye to the host, who didn't see me. I walked out knowing I would never be such a fool again.

Whilst we're chatting about people pleasing, I want to have a word about toxic people, a bit like the ones at the party to be honest. These people drag our self-esteem down further.

Toxic people will try and manipulate you and change you for their own gains, so you keep them happy whilst ignoring your happiness. Sometimes, without realising what we're doing, we associate with them because it affirms our belief that we're unworthy, so when they treat us badly you think, 'Well, of course they do, I'm a bad person'.

You might stay with these people because you think that no one else will like you.

At other times a part of us is trying to prove to them that we *are* worthy. It's complicated but the bottom line is if you're constantly altering yourself to meet other people's expectations, then you're not being you and not thinking of you.

We need tight boundaries to make sure we're protected. We have to learn the art of saying no. We have to cultivate friendships based on mutual respect, honesty and self-awareness. The people that use us, but don't see us, can go to hell.

By the way, an interesting byproduct of liking yourself is attracting others. People are drawn towards confidence and self-assurance. I'm not saying this should be your only motivation to sort your self-esteem, but just know that good things come when we value ourselves.

When we stand up for what we want and what we believe, our self-esteem starts to blossom.

36. Be more trainspotter

I've joined a book group. I'm quite a book nerd, it has to be said. I can talk full pelt on the joys of *I Capture the Castle* or *The Enchanted April* or *84 Charing Cross Road* or the *Cazalet Chronicles* or *If Morning Ever Comes* or *The Night Watch* or ... actually, I'll stop now, but I think you understand my passion.

I've come to the group prepared, having read *The Handmaid's Tale* (very good it was, too; you should read it) and I'm ready to go. We talk about what we thought about the book and then start to discuss the other books we love.

It's a great conversation, people rhapsodising about the darkness of *Jane Eyre* or the intensity of *The Joy Luck Club*. We shriek with disagreement: 'What? You actually managed to finish *Ulysses*? I couldn't get past the first paragraph!' 'Really? You're telling me you liked *One Hundred Years of Solitude*? I thought it was terrible.' There's universal agreement on *Pride and Prejudice* and only one dissenting voice on *The Catcher in the Rye*. I decide never to talk to them again, ever, ever because it's such a great book.

The whole meeting gives me a surge of energy and, when I cycle back home, I realise how great I'm feeling about myself. And it's because I feel seen. Because I feel validated.

I always felt like the weird kid at school who loved books when all my friends were into cars or football or hardstyle psychedelic trance music. I was desperate to connect to others who got as excited as I did about a line from a WH Auden poem or the new short-story collection from Alice Munro.

Similarly, I did an art history evening course and was fizzing when we covered Amedeo Modigliani, Mark Rothko and Gwen John. Now, you may have never heard of these artists but for me it was joyous hearing how other people loved them too; it was like finding my own tribe.

When we're with our people, there is a fizz in the room, an infectious energy that fuels your self-esteem. It could be crochet, baking or collecting photos of hedgehogs. You might adore watching videos of foxes feasting from bins or salsa dancing. Your passion for your passions is a fantastic thing.

People who make fun of trainspotters have no idea how good they feel about themselves because they're pursuing something they love. Whenever I see them at the end of the platform writing down the number of a train, or waiting for the next locomotive to arrive, it gives me a thrill to see them so happy.

When we're with the people we connect to, we feel great about ourselves. When we pursue what we love, we feel great about ourselves.

Find your people, your places, your things and see your self-esteem grow.

149

37. Laugh at your thoughts

I'm supposed to be meeting my friend to go to the cinema, but the bus I'm on has broken down in the middle of countryside. I'm really annoyed with myself, despite it not being my fault and there being nothing I can do about it until a replacement arrives. And then comes the negative self-esteem thoughts.

'You should have left earlier, you imbecile.'

'This has happened because you're a disorganised mess.'

'What an idiot you are, always making these mistakes.'

I call my friend and explain what's happened, they completely understand, but still the voice persists.

'You've let him down; what a bad friend you are.'

'If you cared about other people, this wouldn't have happened.'

Once the thoughts are let loose, they keep coming and coming. We missed the film and went to another one instead, but the whole time my brain kept chastising me.

When I got home, I realised that I couldn't keep going like this, I had to get control of my thoughts. Which is when I invented Sir Henry.

I want you to picture a private members club in London. There are wood-panelled walls, low level lamps, people reading newspapers and a string of servants tending to the members' needs. A man of a certain age is sat in a red leather wingback, drinking a very expensive single malt whisky. It looks as though he has maybe had a few already.

151

This is Sir Henry Pissinger and, to be honest, I probably have nothing in common with him at all, but he's really, really good at laughing at his self-esteem thoughts so I use him all the time to help with mine.

Sir Henry uses laughter to tackle his unwanted thoughts because he knows you can't help a thought, but you can help your reaction to it.

He cackles, he chortles and he doesn't let the thoughts get to him. If he hears, 'You are useless, Sir Henry, a monstrous terrible person,'
he responds by chortling,
'What poppycock, what
nonsense, what piff paff,
what utterly jelly-filled
ludicrosity. Now, go on,
piss off.'

If he hears a voice

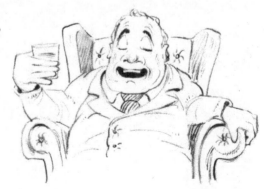

saying, 'You, Sir Henry, have achieved nothing with your life,' he sniggers with glee, he positively guffaws. 'What gibberish, what hogwash, what balderdash, now poo off, you dried lizard penis.'

I love this reaction to unwanted self-esteem thoughts, it's exactly how we should treat them, with the contempt they deserve. You see, if we let the thoughts have room in our brain, they will grow and fester. If we quickly whack them, tell them to 'do one', we aren't reacting to the negativity and we stop the spiralling.

When we use Sir Henry's reaction, we're saying, 'This is just a thought, that's all it is and I won't entertain such claptrap.' The thought pings off from your brain into oblivion.

You can repeat this process whenever a low self-esteem thought comes. The thought is much shorter-lived, and you can get on with your life. It's like having a laughter forcefield; the thought comes in and is repelled.

38. I sausage work harder

Damn it, I should be a better person.

I should be cleverer. I should be better with money. I should be richer. I should be kinder. I should be more attractive. I should be fitter. I should be more successful. I should work harder. I should be more motivated. I should be more fun. I should be a better husband. I should be a better son. I should be a better parent. You can fill in the blanks yourself in case I've missed anything off the list.

Using the word 'should' in any sentence relating to yourself is bad news for your self-esteem. 'Should' tells us we aren't doing well enough, that we need to try harder, that we're doing badly. The word places emphasis on failure rather than progress.

I was once giving a talk about self-esteem to quite a large group of people. They seemed like a nice bunch – someone even complimented my striped braces, which is always good in my book. I was explaining the importance of not using the word should and someone heckled, 'What a load of bloody nonsense, you're a total idiot, it's just a word, changing your vocabulary can't make a difference to your self-esteem.'

Had I magically transported myself into a subterranean comedy club? Was I doing thirty minutes of satirical stand up in front of an inebriated crowd?

I replied, 'Well, that's where you're wrong, mister, and if you know everything about self-esteem why are you at this talk?' Okay, I didn't actually say that, instead I blew a large raspberry in his face and stuck my tongue out. Okay, I did neither of these things but I really, really wanted to.

What I did was wait until the end of the talk and then I tackled his comment. I explained that words have a lot of power. The word 'should' has more power than others.

Take the word 'sausage', for example. 'Should' is definitely a more powerful word than 'sausage'. If we replace the word 'should' with 'sausage', we totally change it:

'I sausage work harder.'

'I sausage be a better person.'

'I sausage be more motivated.'

It just sounds like a sausage has come to life and is struggling with the English language.

To make the adjustment to not using should, we initially change 'should' to 'I'd like to'. Then it's much less harsh and judgemental.

'I'd like to work harder.'

'I'd like to be a better person.'

'I'd like to be more motivated.'

Sounds much better, doesn't it? Stick with that for a while and then you can assess whether the thought is something that you genuinely want to improve or whether it's coming from a place of low self-esteem.

You see, I often want to be a better person, I want to be kinder to people and I think that's a good thing to work towards. It comes from a place of improvement, not self-criticism – so I stick to 'I'd like to'. But with 'I should be more attractive' I remove the should altogether because it's just a product of my low self-esteem. See the difference?

I remember not to use should with this little rhyme thingy, **should equals bad wood** – because the word is useless, it does nothing for our self-esteem. Put bad wood on a fire and it's not going to burn and that's what we want to do with your self-esteem, make it grow, make it bright, make it ignite.

155

39. Do more things by yourself

I have to get across London, which never goes well.

If I'm with my husband Patrick, I just follow him because he lived there for a long time and can navigate his way around the city using some kind of inbuilt intuitive satnav. He goes down alleys that seem to appear from nowhere and then declares it will be much quicker if we 'just nip through St Paul's Cathedral'. But he's not coming away with me and I have to figure out how to get the train, the underground, hire a black cab, get a ferry, jog across Hyde Park, take a swan pedalo, rent a bike and then mount a passing shire horse.

I have no sense of direction. Seriously, I mean none. This isn't false modesty. Once when I was in Paris with some friends, I agreed to do the directions which said go north, so I headed up some steps because up a hill to me is north and going down a hill is south. After forty-five minutes and ending up in a less than salubrious area of the city, my mates realised what I was doing. They banned

me from ever doing the directions again. We got a taxi
to where we were supposed to be in the first place. I paid
for all the drinks that night. And the next night. And the
following night.

Anyway, I have planned my route with precision. I have
paper copies of what I have to do, it's all on my phone in my
electronic notes and I've emailed it to myself too. Patrick
is poised on his phone in case I need emergency support.
He's basically the fourth emergency service and is avail-
able at very reasonable rates in case you need urgent
London-based directions.

The first train arrives on time. Tick. I nearly head down
the escalators to the wrong line of the underground but
catch myself and get the right way – another tick. I walk
about seven hundred miles to get to the correct platform,
nearly going the wrong way but I correct myself – tick,
tick, tick. Then I have to navigate a few streets to the next
train station. I use my phone and get there unscathed –
tick. There is a brief interlude when I move one way to let
someone pass, they go the same way, I move the other way,
they do the same and we do this dance for some consider-
able time.

I eventually get to the other side of London and release
several party poppers and a sequence of multi-coloured
firecrackers to celebrate. I haven't needed help from
Patrick, I haven't had to phone the police, I haven't handed

myself in to the lost property office at Paddington station. I've done well.

You might be thinking, 'For goodness' sake, you've only got yourself across London. What do you want, a trophy?' Well, yes, a trophy would be very nice please. For me, this is big and I'm proud of myself.

I encourage you to do loads of independent stuff as well, because doing things by yourself has a far-reaching impact on your self-esteem and confidence. It gives you proof that you can achieve things on your own, without the help of others.

You don't need to be taking on anything massive like scaling the Eiffel Tower using elastic bands or ski-dooing across a partially frozen Lake Geneva. I mean, you can do these things if you want, and they'll definitely be good for your self-worth but you may also die and that kind of puts a dampener on the self-esteem thing we're trying to do here.

What's important is that you do it and remember the good feeling it gives you.

I want you to write all these things down, on your phone, on some paper – hell, you can spell it out in Lego if you want (actually, that would be kind of cool – please do that). Record it and when you're feeling crap about yourself you've got a fantastic list of stuff you did.

I don't care if you're thirteen and you've just landed your first Saturday job or you're ninety-five and have just completed your first zoom call to your grandchildren in New Zealand – it all matters, it all counts because independent acts lead to independent thinking, which in turn leads to increased self-worth.

We change a wheel on our bike by ourselves, bake some bread, get a plant to grow, get up and do karaoke or ... get across London, it's all proof that we're capable and worthy and absolutely friggin' awesome.

159

40. Be your own sweet, weird self

I'm going out to dinner with a friend and some of her
mates, who I haven't met before. I'm sat on my bed trying
to work out what I can wear to give the impression that
I'm a sophisticated man about town, when in fact I haven't
been out to dinner in months and think I may have worn
the same socks for three days running.

I phone my friend Mitch who I turn to during existen-
tial fashion crises.

> MITCH: Well, what do you want to wear?
>
> ME: I don't know, that's why I'm phoning you.
>
> MITCH: What are the options?
>
> ME: I could wear my blue trousers, blue top and blue
> t-shirt.
>
> MITCH: Do you want to look like a blueberry?
>
> ME: Possibly.

MITCH: Is it a fruit-based gathering? Will other people be dressed as pomegranates?

ME: I don't know.

MITCH: You should dress as you.

ME: I think that's a bad idea.

MITCH: Why?

ME: Because . . . well, I don't want to stand out.

MITCH: Again, why?

ME: Because people might judge me.

MITCH: What if they do?

ME: I guess. I really want to wear my green trousers, red braces, flowery shirt, my wooden bangle and my tweed cap.

MITCH: Then do it! Look, it's way more important to be you than worry about what some random person who you won't meet again is thinking about you over dinner.

161

I wore the outfit and felt great, not only because I made the right decision, and someone said they liked my cap, but mostly because I was myself. Being yourself is absolutely key to raising and maintaining your self-esteem.

As long as you're not hurting or deliberately offending others, make every effort to be your authentic self. When we're ourselves the message we send ourselves is 'I'm worthy and it's okay to be who I am.' Every time you **don't** make a concession based on fear, it becomes a big tick for your self-esteem.

You have to wear what you want. If that's a purple and cerise tutu, partnered with a hyacinth bikini top and sparkly black boots, then go for it. Few things bring me as much joy as seeing people who don't concede to their fears of being judged. People who re-enact the Battle of Waterloo wearing full military regalia. People who dance in the hills on a spring morning with their French poodles. People who swim in the sea with no care about what others think of their body. It's pure freedom and the freedom is being you.

Avoidance and conformity only feed low self-esteem. When our self-esteem is low, the tendency is to avoid situations where we might feel judged and people who might judge us. We hide ourselves away in clothes that cover us up or wear things that won't get noticed. We don't do things for fear that people will think we're 'odd'.

Oddness is a beautiful, beautiful thing, people – it's not strange, it's stunning and so are you.

Secret summary

Ahoy there! Here is a bonus chapter of sorts. I thought it would be useful to offer a bit of a summary that you can look at quickly when you need a reminder – a sort of self-esteem boost if you will.

* Make a list of your good bits
* Don't care as much about what people think
* Do some meaningful activity
* Tell yourself you're alright
* Be okay with making mistakes
* Don't compare yourself to other people
* Don't avoid, don't procrastinate
* Don't believe the people who said you were bad
* Have compassion for yourself
* Rely on you not other people
* Take your low self-esteem to court – what's the evidence?
* Do uncomfortable things

* Forgive yourself for past mistakes
* Change your core beliefs to more realistic ones
* Don't catastrophise
* Celebrate your achievements
* Take care of emotional and physical health
* Realise how ludicrous your negative self-talk is
* Don't use crutches to raise your esteem
* Use the word 'but' in sentences to take the power out of your negative self-talk
* Hating yourself is not the solution to your low self-esteem
* Name it, frame it then reframe it
* Create an imaginary confident friend
* Write down things you're thankful for
* Don't say things to yourself that you wouldn't say to a friend
* Ask for what you want
* Get some perspective on life
* Learn to laugh at yourself
* Catch your automatic self-hating remarks
* Ask for feedback about yourself from friends
* Have more childlike fun
* Stay within your moral code
* Get angry with your negative self-talk
* You are valid no matter how you feel about your physical appearance

* Stop people pleasing
* Find your passions and the people that share them
* Laugh at your self-esteem thoughts
* Never use the word 'should'
* Do more things by yourself
* Be weird, be yourself

Finally, remember, you are enough, you are important and have a place in this world.

Acknowledgements

166   Thank you to Tom Asker and all at Robinson.
As always, thank you to Patrick.